RECENT VIEWS ON HYPERTROPHIC CARDIOMYOPATHY

DEVELOPMENTS IN CARDIOVASCULAR MEDICINE

RECENT VIEWS ON HYPERTROPHIC CARDIOMYOPATHY

edited by

E. VAN DER WALL and K.I. LIE

Department of Cardiology
Groningen University Hospital
Groningen
The Netherlands

1985 **MARTINUS NIJHOFF PUBLISHERS**
a member of the KLUWER ACADEMIC PUBLISHERS GROUP
BOSTON / DORDRECHT / LANCASTER

Distributors

for the United States and Canada: Kluwer Academic Publishers, 190 Old Derby Street, Hingham, MA 02043, USA
for the UK and Ireland: Kluwer Academic Publishers, MTP Press Limited, Falcon House, Queen Square, Lancaster LA1 1RN, UK
for all other countries: Kluwer Academic Publishers Group, Distribution Center, P.O. Box 322, 3300 AH Dordrecht, The Netherlands

Library of Congress Cataloging in Publication Data

Recent views on hypertrophic cardiomyopathy.

  (Developments in cardiovascular medicine)
  Papers presented at a symposium held July 6th, 1984
at the University Hospital Groningen.
  Bibliography: p.
  Includes index.
  1. Heart--Hypertrophy--Congresses. I. Wall, E.,
van der. II. Lie, K. I. III. Series.
RC685.H9R43 1985   616.1'2   84-25419

ISBN-13: 978-94-010-8711-7   e-ISBN-13: 978-94-009-4994-2
DOI: 10.1007/978-94-009-4994-2

Copyright

Contents

VI

Preface

In Groningen there has been a continuous investigation of hypertrophic cardio-myopathy for almost twenty years. Members of this working-group have tried to study the many aspects of this intriguing disease, and it is in this volume that they present their recent results and current concepts (chapters 2, 3, 5 and 6). A contribution from the Dutch interuniversity Institute of Cardiology presenting a detailed account of evaluation by means of radionuclide techniques completes the non-invasive picture of cardiomyopathies (chapter 4).

On July 6th, 1984, a symposium entitled 'Recent views on hypertrophic cardio-myopathy' was held at the University Hospital Groningen. The main reason to organize this meeting was the retirement of one of our working-group members, namely E. van der Wall, as head of the cardiological department. The speakers at the symposium presented their lectures based on their contributions to this book. It is an honour for us to have obtained their full cooperation for this book and for the symposium.

We are very grateful that this Groningen manifestation could include the outstanding contributions of several well-known experts from abroad. We there-fore thank our colleagues Profs. Epstein, Goodwin, Kaltenbach and Schulte for their spontaneous and valuable cooperation (chapters 1, 7, 8 and 9). Thanks to their efforts especially, this book has acquired the international character that the study of this subject deserves.

It will be evident to the reader that the different contributions reflect different opinions, a fact we hope will promote rather than disturb the flexibility in approach to the various and variable problems of this particular disorder.

The generous help of Knoll BV, The Netherlands, is very gratefully acknowl-edged. Without their assistance this book would not have been published.

Groningen, July 1984   E. van der Wall and K.I. Lie

List of contributors

Blanksma, P.K.
Department of Cardiology, Groningen University Hospital, Oostersingel 59, 9713 EZ Groningen, The Netherlands

Bircks, W.
Department of Thoracic and Cardiovascular Surgery, University of Düsseldorf, Surgical Clinic B, Moorenstrasse 5, D-4000 Düsseldorf, FRG

Bonow, R.O.
Cardiology Branch, Building 10, National Heart, Lung and Blood Institute, Bethesda MD 20205, USA

Cannon III, R.O.
Cardiology Branch, Building 10, National Heart, Lung and Blood Institute, Bethesda MD 20205, USA.

Epstein .S.E.
Cardiology Branch, Building 10, National Heart, Lung and Blood Institute, Bethesda MD 20205, USA

Goodwin J.F.
Royal Postgraduate Medical School, Ducane Road, London W12 OHS, UK

Hamer, J.P.M.
Department of Cardiology, Groningen University Hospital, Oostersingel 59, 9713 EZ Groningen, The Netherlands

Hopf, R.
Department of Cardiology, Medical Clinic, Wolfgang von Goethe University, Theodor Stern Kai 7, D-6000 Frankfort, FRG

Kaltenbach, M.
  Department of Cardiology, Medical Clinic, Wolfgang von Goethe University,
  Theodor Stern Kai 7, D-6000 Frankfurt, FRG

Lie, K.I.
  Department of Cardiology, Groningen University Hospital, Oostersingel 59,
  9713 EZ Groningen, The Netherlands

Maron, B.J.
  Cardiology Branch, Building 10, National Heart, Lung and Blood Institute,
  Bethesda MD 20205, USA

Rosing D.R.
  Cardiology Branch, Building 10, National Heart, Lung and Blood Institute,
  Bethesda MD 20205, USA

Schulte, H.D.
  Department of Thoracic and Cardiovascular Surgery, University of Düsseldorf, Surgical Clinic B, Moorenstrasse 5, D-4000 Düsseldorf, FRG

Van der Wall, E.
  Department of Cardiology, Groningen University Hospital, Oostersingel 59,
  9713 EZ Groningen, The Netherlands

Van der Wall, E.E.
  Interuniversity Institute of Cardiology, Free University Hospital, De Boele-
  laan 1117, 1081 HV Amsterdam, The Netherlands

Van Veldhuisen, D.J.
  Department of Cardiology, Groningen University Hospital, Oostersingel 59,
  9713 EZ Groningen, The Netherlands

Viersma, J.W.
  Department of Cardiology, Groningen University Hospital, Oostersingel 59,
  9713 EZ Groningen, The Netherlands

1. Recent views on hypertrophic cardiomyopathy

J.F. GOODWIN

The current approaches to hypertrophic cariomyopathy involve three main areas: the continuing debate on 'obstruction', the natural history, and methods of management. There is general, though not universal, agreement that hypertrophic cardiomyopathy is a distinct disease entity, albeit with many different aspects and a spectrum of features.

The problem of 'obstruction'

Traditionally, over the last two to three decades, hypertrophic cardiomyopathy has been regarded first as a purely outflow tract obstructive disorder, and then later as a condition in which obstruction might or might not be present so that a so-called 'non-obstructive' type was described. Despite the challenge twenty years ago that 'obstruction' was not a true feature, the view that gradients indicated mechanical obstruction, and that this was an important feature of the disease, still holds the minds of many experts in the field. Others maintain that gradients are evidence of catheter entrapment [1], of intraventricular compression, and are signs of a powerful hypertrophic muscle rather than a true obstruction to outflow. Where does the truth lie? Like most opposing theories, there is probably some truth in both.

Reasons for considering the gradients to be dynamic rather than obstructive can be stated as follows:

1. There is no relation between gradients on the one hand and prognosis and symptoms on the other. Gradients tend to disappear as the disease advances [2].
2. Gradients are extremely labile and can vary from zero to 100 mHg or more.
3. The contents of the left ventricle are expelled rapidly in the first half to two thirds of systole.
4. The ejection fraction is usually high–up to 90% in many patients, confirming complete emptying of the left ventricle.

5. Flow studies show that aortic flow velocity may actually be increased when gradients develop under positive inotropic stimulation [3].

Recent work in the department of Clinical Cardiology at the Royal Postgraduate Medical School has revealed that the rapid ejection of the contents of the left ventricle in the first two thirds of systole is identical both in patients with gradients and in those without, denying the importance of true obstruction.

I have suggested [4] that the gradients are produced by elimination of the ventricular cavity by the powerful contractions of the greatly hypertrophied ventricular muscle. The mid portion and apex of the left ventricle are cut off from the outflow tract as the powerful contraction squeezes the cavity away. By then, however, the contents of the left ventricle have been largely or completely expelled.

On the other hand, there is some support for the view that obstruction to outflow is a basic characteristic of the disease, and not an incidental occurrence, and that subgroups can be detected. These are: muscular subaortic stenosis; latent muscular subaortic stenosis; non-obstructive hypertrophic cardiomyopathy; mid-ventricular obstruction and asymmetrical septal hypertrophy [5]. Different patterns of left ventricular ejection are claimed for the different subgroups [6], while Morgan et al. [7]and Ross et al. [8] have suggested that in the presence of an obstructive pressure gradient 70% of left ventricular ejection occurs in the presence of the gradient and thereby produces a significant systolic overload and prolongation of ejection time [9].

The weight of evidence would seem to suggest that, systolic anterior motion and mitral-septal contact notwithstanding, true obstruction is not a reality in most cases of hypertrophic cardiomyopathy. There may well be some patients in whom hypertrophy is massive and the ventricular cavity extremely small so that papillary muscle overgrowth genuinely blocks the cavity and obstructs outflow.

There is, in my view, no reason to suppose that different sites of hypertrophy of the septum denote different types of the disease; hypertrophy may be symmetrical or asymmetrical, and if the former, can affect the upper, middle or distal portions of the septum. The site of the asymmetrical hypertrophy may influence the angiocardiographic and echocardiographic appearances of the ventricle, and occasionally even the electrocardiogram, which may show deep T wave inversion in the apical portion of the septum involved.

The natural history of prognosis

The experience at Hammersmith Hospital and Royal Postgraduate Medical School and from other sources indicates that sudden death occurs in around 13% of patients. Of 254 patients followed for from 1–23 years, 58 died; 33 suddenly [10]. The worst prognosis is in young patients with symptoms who have a family history of sudden death [11, 12]. The average annual mortality for all patients is around 2.6%, but in the high risk group it is double.

Other modes of death are congestive heart failure, infective endocarditis and its complications, and severe mitral regurgitation.

The causes of sudden death are both 'electrical' and 'mechanical'. The commonest cause is electrical and is due to ventricular arrhythmia. Ambulant electrocardiographic monitoring has shown serious ventricular arrhythmias (multiform frequent ventricular premature contractions and runs of ventricular tachycardia) in one third of patients. These episodes are usually asymptomatic and may occur at any time. There is a significant relation between such arrhytmias and sudden death. Occasionally accessory pathways between atria and ventricle may lead to fatal arrhytmias [13]. The onset of atrial fibrillation, while not in itself usually fatal, may lead to very serious haemodynamic disturbance owing to the loss of atrial drive and the shortened filling time for the left ventricle caused by the rapid heart rate.

The mechanical causes of sudden death result mainly from diastolic ventricular faults. The stiff inelastic left ventricle, with its reduced compliance and impaired global and regional relaxation, cannot fill adequately in the presence of tachycardia or atrial fibrillation. Impaired filling reduces heart volume and increases the elimination of the left ventricle by the partially contracted hypertrophied wall. Thus the passage of blood through the heart is halted, coronary flow falls disastrously, and syncope or death results from terminal ventricular fibrillation. We have reported such a case [14].

There may be some connection between arrhythmic death and sudden death due to diastolic dysfunction in that an echocardiographic study at the Royal Postgraduate Medical School showed that patients with ventricular tachycardia had severely impaired septal motion [15].

Management of hypertrophic cardiomyopathy

Management should be directed towards the prevention of arrhythmia, and improvement in diastolic function. Naturally, it is desirable to prevent the progression of the disease, but at the present time, there is no certain method of doing this.

Treatment must also be directed towards complications, such as atrial fibrillation, congestive heart failure, infective endocarditis, mitral regurgitation, and bradycardia. It is apparent that the practice of using beta blockade (or calcium channel blockade) on a routine basis for all patients without systolic pressure gradients while employing septal resection for those with gradients, is no longer tenable. Treatment must be tailored to the needs of indiviudal patients, bearing in mind the abnormalities underlying the disease.

Regular observations

Follow-up is essential in order to monitor treatment and to note changes in the pattern of the disease.

The most important follow-up examination is ambulatory electrocardiographic monitoring to detect arrhythmias. Twenty-four, or preferably forty–eight, hour monitoring should be carried out at yearly intervals in patients without symptoms or family history of sudden death who have not shown arrhythmias on the initial study. Those who have a family history of sudden death or symptoms, require monitoring at six monthly intervals. All patients should be urged to report any new symptoms or changes at once.

Patients who have no symptoms, no family history of sudden death, mild disease, and no arrhythmias need not receive any medicines, but of course must be regularly checked. Those who have been demonstrated to have frequent or multiform premature ventricular contractions or runs of ventricular tachycardia should be given amiodarone and checked regularly by monitoring, and also by liver function tests and thyroid function tests. Chest radiographs are necessarey regularly to detect any sign of pulmonary fibrosis. This last is the most serious side–effect of amiodarone, and any respiratory symptoms should be carefully investigated. Slit lamp examination for corneal deposits is necessary every six months or so. Symptoms are dose-related, so therefore the dose of amiodarone should be kept as low as possible: 600 mgm daily for 5 days loading dose, then 400 mgm daily for maintenance dose each week. In some patients, 200 mgm daily may suffice.

Patients who have symptoms (angina, dyspnoea, dizziness) require treatment in order to improve diastolic function. The approach of choice remains beta blockade with propranolol, but this does not always improve diastolic function or relieves symptoms [15a, 16]. Better drugs are needed, and possibly calcium channel blocking agents may represent an improvement on beta adrenergic blockade.

Verapamil has been shown to relieve symptoms, reduce gradients and improve exercise tolerance [17, 18]. However, it has potentially serious complications: sudden death and pulmonary oedema [19]. It should not be used if there is any conduction defect or if the pulmonary venous wedge pressure is high. Verapamil should be given cautiously, started in hospital using small doses of 20 mgm three times daily initially, with careful checking for signs of pulmonary congestion or development of conduction defects.

Recent work suggests that verapamil may exert a beneficial effect on diastolic function [20], but the results may be variable and paradoxical [21]. Most recently, Anderson et al. [22] have shown that left ventricular total systolic volume index and end–diastolic volume index increase without any significant change in left ventricular end–diastolic pressure. This suggests improved diastolic function.

Lorell et al. [23] have shown that the calcium channel blocking agent, nifedipine, improves diastolic function. The vasodilator action of nifedipine is potentially dangerous by reducing left ventricular volume, but the benefits gained from improved diastolic filling may outweigh the dangers. More work is necessary on nifedipine in hypertrophic cardiomyopathy, but it may be tried cautiously in hospital, starting with small doses of not more than 10 mgm three times daily with careful checks of blood pressure.

Patients with both symptoms and arrhythmia need a combination of drugs for left ventricular compliance and for arrhythmia. Amiodarone may be combined with propranolol but should not be used with verapamil. Its use with nifedipine has yet to be studied and validated. An alternative approach is the use of sotalol which has an action similar to amiodarone and also a beta blocking effect. Preliminary experience suggests some benefit, but less effect on symptoms than propranolol.

In patients with syncope as a prominent feature, it may be difficult to determine whether arrhythmia or diastolic fault is responsible. An effort test may help by showing arrhythmia, or by producing symptoms and hypotension, suggesting impaired filling of the heart.

When the outflow gradient is more than 50 Hg and persists, and when there are symptoms that are intractable to medicines, septal resection may be considered if there is marked asymmetrical hypertrophy. Septal resection may be expected to relieve symptoms and gradients, but not to alter prognosis favourably. It should be regarded essentially as a procedure only for relief of symptoms. Unfortunately, the mortality of the operation is not negligible.

Treatment of complications

Atrial fibrillation. The onset of rapid atrial fibrillation should be regarded as a medical emergency. Embolism is a hazard, and the patient should be given anticoagulants at once – initially heparin and then warfarin. Cardioversion should be carried out as soon as possible. Cardioversion may be potentiated by the use of amiodarone. Large doses by mouth (800–1000 mgm per day) for two days may achieve an adequate tissue level, or if less urgency, 600 mgm daily may be given for 5–7 days prior to cardioversion. Amiodarone itself may achieve cardioversion of stabilise the arrhythmia. Intravenous amiodarone may have an erratic action and is not recommended for routine use. Digitalis may be used to control ventricular rate if necessary, but its effect is potentiated by amiodarone.

Congestive heart failure. Congestive heart failure usually indicated that the disease process has become widespread throughout the ventricular muscle and denotes a late stage at which systolic pump failure is added to diastolic failure. Treatment is extremely difficult. Often a gradient, previously present, disappears, and with it the typical murmur [2]. Gradients and murmurs may persist, however, and if a loud systolic murmur is heard the possibility of serious mitral regurgitation having developed, and being responsible for the heart failure must be carefully considered and further investigated.

The treatment of congestive heart failure is essentially along conventional lines, bearing in mind that vasodilators are contraindicated, and beta blockade and verapamil should be avoided. Diuretics are needed but digitalis should not be used unless essential to control ventricular rate in atrial fibrillation. Amiodarone is not contra-indicated, and is valuable to control atrial fibrillation. The case for nifedipine in patients with heart failure is not yet decided.

Infective endocarditis. Infection, when it strikes, nearly always involves the mitral valve. Treatment is exactly as for other forms of infective endocarditis in other heart situations, bearing in mind that surgical treatment may be required. Early diagnosis is vital for successful treatment.

Mitral regurgitation. Mitral regurgitation is present in minor degree in all patients with gradients, and is not of therapeutic significance. However, in a small minority of patients, the mitral valve is virtually destroyed by calcification or infection, and extreme mitral regurgitation results. This causes severe dyspnoea or even pulmonary oedema and modifies the clinical signs of the underlying disease: the systolic murmur becomes full length, a short decrescendo mitral diastolic murmur develops, and calcification may be detected on the mitral valve by echocardiography or radiography. The diagnosis from rheumatic heart disease may become impossible clinically, especially if there is atrial fibrillation (unless ther is a very suggestive history), and the true condition may only emerge after echocardiography or, more likely, angiocardiography.

Treatment is by mitral valve replacement, using either a bioprosthesis or a low profile disc valve, since the left ventricular cavity is usually too small to accept a ball valve prosthesis.

Bradycardia. The place of pacemakers in the treatment of hypertrophic cardiomyopathy is not yet fully defined.

A pacemaker may be considered when useful beta blocking therapy to relieve symptoms causes unacceptable or dangerous bradycardia. Moreover, some patients have conduction defects, complete heart block or sinus node disease, necessitating pacemaking.

Conventional pacemakers have the disadvantage of removing atrial drive in patients with sinus bradycardia or first or second degree heart block.

Newer generations of sequential pacemakers may be expected to make a contribution to the treatment of hypertrophic cardiomyopathy.

References

1. Criley JM, Lewis KB, White RI Jr, Ross RS: Pressure gradients without obstruction: a new concept of hypertrophic subaortic stenosis. Circulation: 32: 881, 1965.
2. Swan DA, Bell B, Oakley CM, Goodwin JF: Analysis of symptomatic course and prognosis and treatment of hypertrophic obstructive cardiomyopathy. Brit Heart J 33: 671, 1971.
3. Murgo JP, Alter BZ, Dorethy JF, Altobelli SA, McGranahan GM: Left ventricular ejection dynamics in hypertrophic cardiomyopathy. In: Sekiguchi M, Olsen EGJ, Cardiomyopathy (eds), University of Tokyo Press, 1980, p 45.
   Goodwin JF: The Frontiers of cardiomyopathy. Brit Heart J 48: 1, 1982.
5. Wigle ED, Rakowski H, Pollick C, Henderson MA, Ruddy TD: Cardiomyopathy: predictions for the foreseeable future. In: Yu PB, Goodwin JF (eds), Lea & Febiger, Philadelphia, 1981 p 185.
6. Bougner DR, Schuld RL, Persaud JA: Hypertrophic obstructive cardiomyopathy – assessment by echocardiographic and Doppler ultrasound. Brit Heart J 37: 917, 1975.
7. Morgan CD, Pollick C, Wigle ED: Cineangiographic timing of left ventricular outflow obstruction and systolic emptying in muscular subaortic stenosis (abstract). Circulation 60 (Suppl I): 262, 1979.
8. Ross J Jr et al.: Mechanics of the intraventricular pressure gradient in idiopathic hypertrophic subaortic stenosis. Circulation 34: 558, 1966.
9. Wigle ED, Auger P, Marquis Y: Muscular subaortic stenosis: the direct relation between intraventricular pressure difference and left ventricular ejection time. Circulation 36: 36, 1967.
10. McKenna WJ et al.: Arrhythmia in hypertrophic cardiomyopathy 1. Influence on prognosis. Brit Heart J 46: 168, 1981.
11. Goodwin JF, Krikler DM: Arrhythmia as a cause of sudden death in hypertrophic cardiomyopathy. Lancet 2: 937, 1976.
12. McKenna WJ, Goodwin JF: The natural history of hypertrophic cardiomyopathy. In: Harvey WP (ed), Current Problems in Cardiology, Vol 6. Chicago/London Year Book Medical Publishers, 1981 p 1.
13. Krikler DM, Davies MJ, Rowland E, Goodwin JF, Evans RC, Shaw DB: Sudden death in hypertrophic cardiomyopathy: associated accessory atrioventricular pathways. Brit Heart J 43: 245, 1980.
14. McKenna WJ, Harris L, Deanfield J: Syncope in hypertrophic cardiomyopathy. Brit Heart J 47: 177, 1982.
15. Doi YL, McKenna WJ, Chetty S, Oakly CM, Goodwin JF: Prediction of mortality and serious ventricular arrhythmia in hypertrophic cardiomyopathy: an echocardiographic study. Brit Heart J 44: 150, 1980.
15a. Hubner PJB, Ziady GM, Lane GK et al.: Double blind trial of propranolol and practolol in hypertrophic cardiomyopathy. Brit Heart J 35: 1116, 1973.
16. Alvares RF, Goodwin JF: Non-invasive assessment of diastolic function in hypertrophic cardiomyopathy on and off beta adrenergic blocking drugs. Brit Heart J 48: 204, 1982.
17. Rosing DR, Kent KM, Borer JS, Seides SF, Maron BJ, Epstein SE: Verapamil therapy: a new approach to the pharmacologic treatment of hypertrophic cardiomyopathy. I Hemodynamic effects. Circulation 60: 1201, 1979.
18. Rosing DR, Kent KM, Maron BJ, Epstein SE: Verapamil therapy: a new approach to the pharmacologic treatment of hypertrophic cardiomyopathy. II. Effects on exercise capacity and symptomatic status. Circulation 60: 1208, 1979.
19. Epstein SE, Rosing DR: Verapamil: its potential for serious complications in patients with hypertrophic cardiomyopathy. Circulation 64: 437, 1981.
20. Bonow RO, Rosing DR, Bacharach SL et al.: Effects of verapamil on left ventricular systolic function and diastolic filling in patients with hypertrophic cardiomyopathy. Circulation 64: 787, 1981.

8

21. Hanrath P, Mathey DG, Kremer P, Sonntag F, Bleifeld W: Effect of verapamil on left ventricular isovolumic relaxation time and regional left ventricular filling in hypertrophic cardiomyopathy. Amer J Cardiol 45: 1258, 1980.
22. Anderson DM, Raff Gl, Ports TA, Brundath BH, Parmley WW, Chatterjee K: Hypertrophic obstructive cardiomyopathy: effects of acute and chronic verapamil treatment on left ventricular systolic and diastolic function. Brit Heart J 51: 523, 1984.
23. Lorell BH, Paulus WJ, Grossman W, Wynne J, Cohn PF: Modification of abnormal left ventricular diastolic properties in patients with hypertrophic cardiomyopathy. Am. J Cardiol 45: 1258, 1982.

2. Problems and pitfalls in the diagnosis of hypertrophic cardiomyopathy by echocardiography

J.P.M. HAMER

With the introduction of echocardiography as a diagnostic aid in the sixties a very important possibility was obtained for the non-invasive visualization of intracardiac structures.

Especially in the first years of the clinical use of this diagnostic tool it was predominantly used for making measurements. It seemed to be possible to measure wall thicknesses, motion patterns and internal diameters and with the time-motion mode even speeds of motion could be determined.

Many investigators at that time tried to find out how useful echocardiography could be for the diagnosis of different cardiac diseases.

The value of echocardiography for the diagnosis of hypertrophic cardiomyopathy (HCM) was first established by Shah [1] and Popp [2]. The thickened interventricular septum (IVS), known from angiocardiographic, surgical and autopsy data, could be recognized on the M-mode echocardiogram in patients with an obstruction of the left ventricular outflow tract. In later years Abbasi [3] also recognized a thickened IVS in patients with an idiopathic HCM without outflow obstruction.

Henry [4] measured the IVS thickness and the thickness of the left ventricular posterior wall (LVPW) or 'free wall' and introduced the septal/free wall ratio. He found that this ratio was more than 1.3 (mean 1.68) in all his patients with asymmetrical septal hypertrophy; with this he added a new name to the dozens of names given to this disorder during the years. He also found this ratio to be independent of the degree of obstruction.

A year later he determined an obstruction index [5] by dividing the duration of outflow narrowing by the mean septal anterior mitral leaflet distance and comparing this with the simultaneously measured peak left ventricular outflow pressure gradient. The duration of narrowing and the narrowing itself, however, were measured with single crystal echocardiography in a selected population with HCM with obstruction.

Rossen [6] studied the degree of systolic thickening and amplitude of excursion of the IVS, also measured with single crystal echocardiography; the septal thickening was significantly reduced from normal as was the septal excursion. Tajik [7] also found a less than normal septal thickening ranging from 0 to 20% which was

30% for normal hearts. The amplitude of excursion was normal in half of his 14 patients, selected to the presence of an obstruction and to a good quality echocardiogram.

The wall thickening of the IVS and LVPW was also measured by Cohen [8]. He also found a hypodynamic IVS and an increase of the contractile capacity of the LVPW with single crystal echocardiography.

In 1975 Henry [9] used one of the first two-dimensional (2-D) systems for the evaluation of obstructive asymmetric septal hypertrophy and found a forward position of the mitral valve in the left ventricular cavity: more insight had been obtained in the spatial anatomy and physiology of the heart.

Measurements were also made from the 2-D image by Cohen [10]; he found a narrowing of the outflow tract in both end-systole and end-diastole. This supported the contention that the anterior leaflet the mitral valve (AML) assumes an abnormally anterior position in idiopathic hypertrophic subaortic stenosis (HCM).

In 1977 Chahine [11] discovered 'no pathognomonic finding in the entity of HCM; it might represent a spectrum of pathology rather than a single well-defined disease'. He investigated 14 patients with single crystal echocardiography.

Until this time, nearly all measurements were made with a single crystal echocardiographic system. This has the disadvantage of lack of spatial orientation, which can easily lead to over- and/or underestimation of wall thicknesses and internal diameters.

We recognized this problem at that time [12] and concluded, in a group of 50 patients with various cardiac diseases investigated with single crystal and 2-D echocardiography, that the position of the heart with respect to the transducer had a great influence on the measurements. This even lead to a false positive diagnosis of HCM on M-mode. Measurements of thickening rates, excursions and thicknesses of the IVS appeared to be very difficult or unreliable without spatial orientation and if the influence of the motion of surrounding cardiac structures could not be visualized.

In 1980 DeMaria [13] concluded with 2-D echocardiography that hypertrophy of the IVS is not uniform from apex to base in all patients but may be the greatest in the apical, mid or basal third: 2-D echocardiography again gave more insight in the anatomic and morphologic features of HCM.

A classical 2-D picture in the long axis view of a basal thickening of the IVS is given in Figures 1 and 2.

More and unusual locations of substantial hypertrophy in patients with HCM were found by Maron and Epstein in 1981 [14, 15, 16] and it appeared to be possible to determine four types of hypertrophy with 2-D echocardiography from the short axis view of the left ventricle at the level of the mitral valve.

The importance of 2-D echocardiography for the diagnosis of HCM was

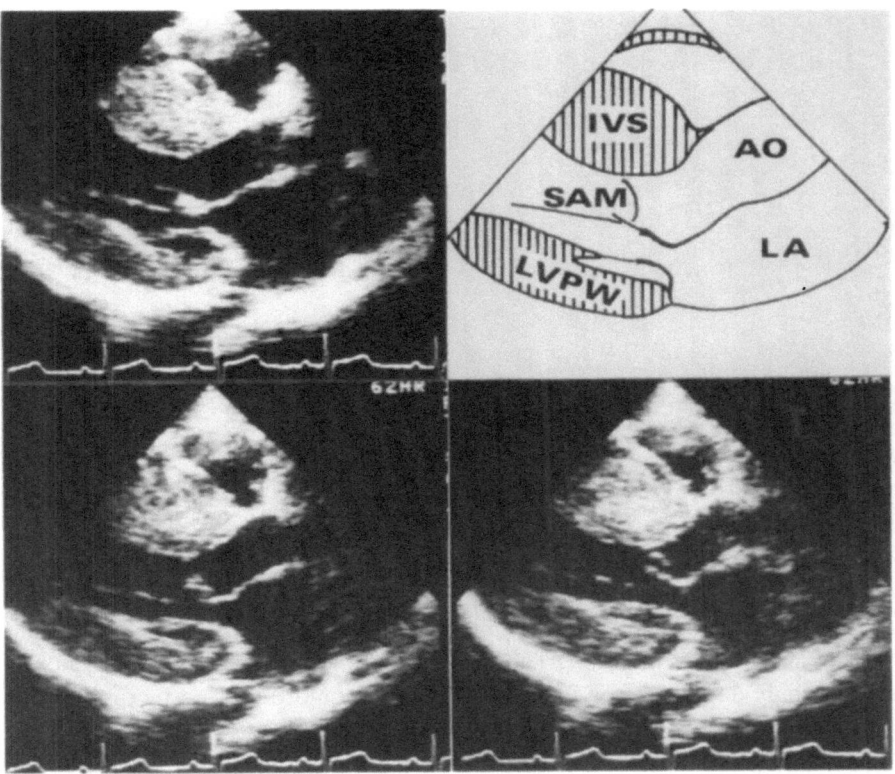

Figure 1. Long axis view of the heart of a 16-year old girl with the classical localization of hypertrophic cardiomyopathy with obstruction. All pictures are made in early systole. There is a discrepancy between the thickness of the interventricular septum (IVS) and the left ventricular posterior wall (LVPW). On the bottom right a systolic anterior motion (SAM) of the mitral apparatus is visualized. The left atrium (LA) is enlarged. AO = aorta.

stressed by Shapiro [17] who also found involvement of various parts of the left ventricle and concluded that only 1 out of 12 patients (from a group of 89 patients) could be correctly diagnosed using M-mode echocardiography.

It may be concluded that until now, 2-D echocardiography has not only been very useful for establishing the diagnosis of HCM but also broadened the concept of this disease: new localizations have been found and different types of cardiomyopathy have been discovered.

However, it is not certain that the limits of echocardiographic diagnosis have been reached. It cannot be excluded that more localizations and less obvious pathologic findings will be discovered.

In this respect it seems reasonable to change the obviously logic question: 'What does echocardiography mean to HCM?' into 'What does HCM mean to echocardiography?'

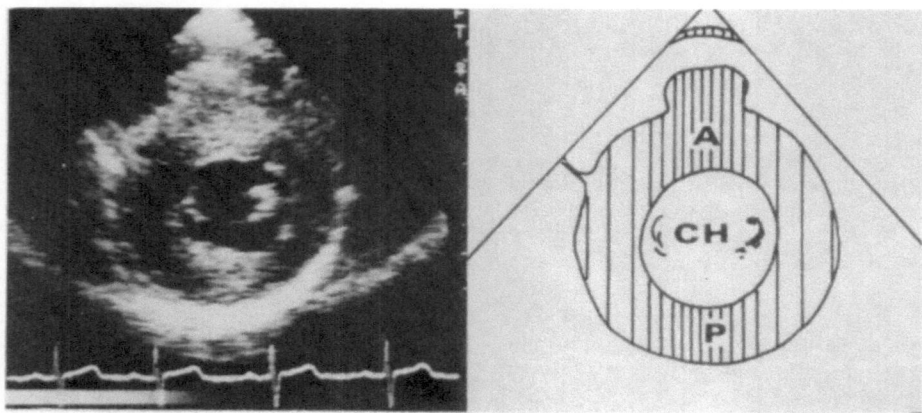

Figure 2. Short axis view of the left ventricle from the same patient as in Figure 1 at the level of the chordae (CH). The anterior part of the left ventricle (A) shows a localized thickening, causing the thickened IVS in Figure 1. The strongest density of the echoes is found in the anterior (A) and posterior part (P) where the sound plane hits the structures more or less perpendicularly, which is also the case in normal left ventricles.

A difference in echo-density might be the consequence of the abnormal microscopical findings in HCM. The conclusion of a difference in density however, is strongly dependent on many factors and should therefore be drawn with great caution; these variables are: the acoustic impedancy of the structure, the distance between transducer and the structure, the gain setting and the angle between the sound beam and the structure (Fig. 2). From our 80 patients with HCM who were echocardiographically revised we have the impression that in several patients a greater echo-density was found from the area involved in HCM (Figs. 3, 6).

A difference in thickness of the area involved in HCM can be found with echocardiography thanks to earlier investigations. This thickened part with respect to the remainder of the ventricle should be compared with normal values and not with other parts of the heart: some parts can be thickened by secondary, 'normal' hypertrophy so that the septal/free wall ratio can be normal in case of HCM as is illustrated in Figure 4. Also, if the sound beam crosses the left ventricle not just below the mitral valve but lower through the papillary muscles, the septal/free wall ratio can be normal as is illustrated in Figure 3.

A difference in thickening rate has also been found from those parts of the ventricle that are involved in HCM.

The consequence of looking for differences is a total echocardiographic screening of both ventricles and a careful measurement of thickness and thickening rates. Thus, it is important to be familiar with the pitfalls that are present in making measurements from M-mode recordings but also with the interpretation of the echocardiogram.

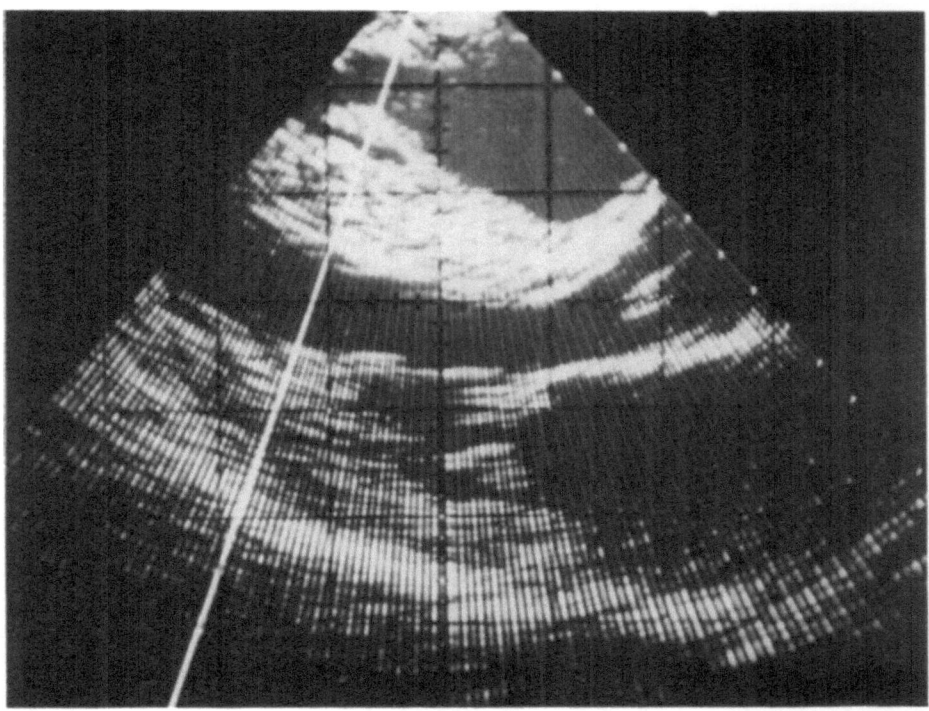

Figure 3. Long axis view of the heart of a patient with hypertrophic cardiomyopathy. The echo-density of the thickened IVS is more than that of the LVPW, which (in a normal gain setting) can be found in a few patients with HCM. The M-mode line crosses the IVS and LVPW too low in the ventricle so that the papillary muscles are included in the M-mode recording, resulting in a wrong interpretation of the thickness of the LVPW. In this case a normal septal/free wall ratio can be measured. For explanation of the figure see Figure 1.

A partial error in the interpretation can be found in the conclusion that the systolic anterior motion (SAM) of part of the mitral apparatus into the outflow tract of the left ventricle is caused by the anterior mitral leaflet. With more experience in echocardiography and improved equipment it can be demonstrated that in many patients with HCM and obstruction, the anterior mitral leaflet remains closed during systole in the presence of a SAM. In those patients the SAM is caused by the chordae (Fig. 4).

From the apical view it can sometimes be seen that even chordae originating from the lateral left ventricular wall can cause a SAM in the absence of mitral regurgitation. This might be due to a shorter distance between the tips of the papillary muscles and the mitral leaflets, resulting in local relatively too long chordae during systole. The Venturi effect in the outflow tract of the left ventricle then sucks the chordae into the direction of the aorta. If this suction is strong enough, a part of the anterior mitral leaflet can also be involved in the SAM. At that

14

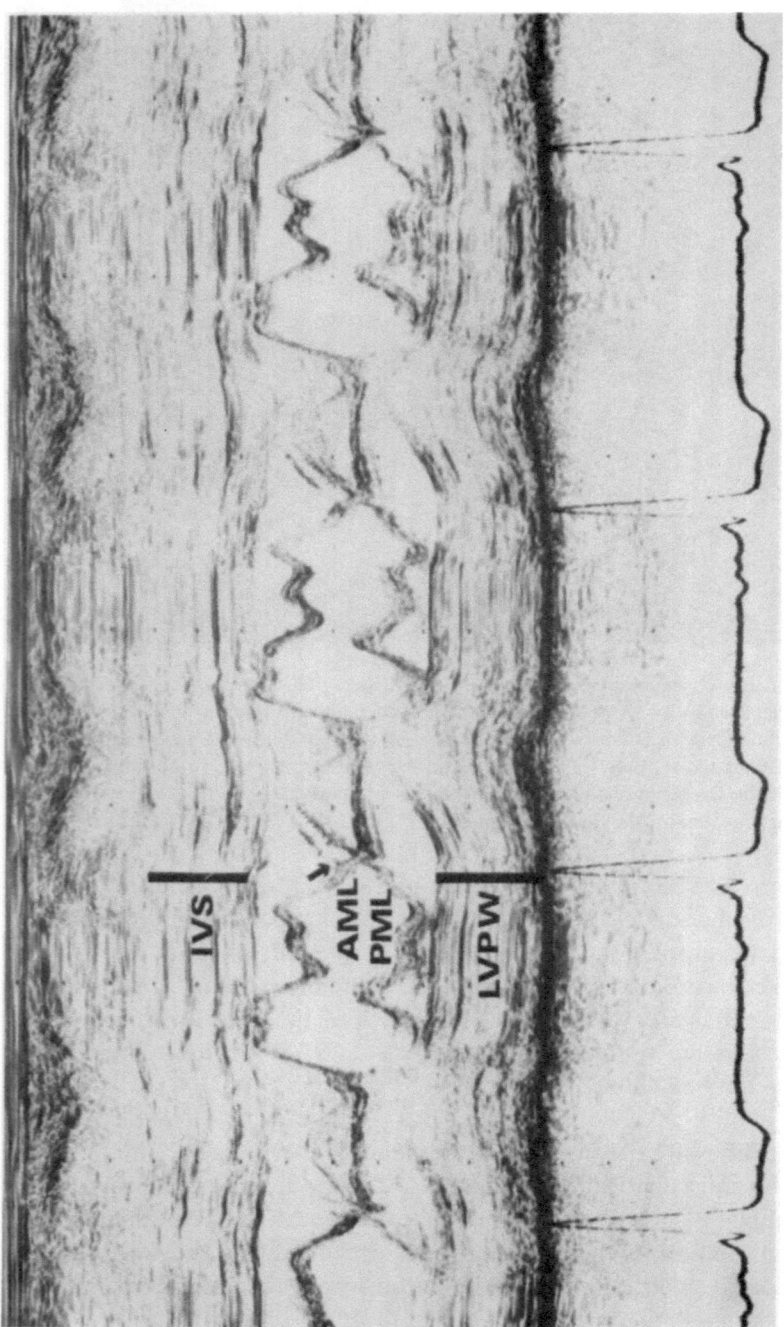

Figure 4. M-mode recording of the heart of a patient with HCM. The IVS is thickened with a diminished thickening rate. However, in this patient a secondary real hypertrophy of the LVPW is found, resulting in a normal septal/free wall ratio. There was no amyloid and no hypertension. A difference is seen between the excursions of the IVS and LVPW, resulting in the diagnosis HCM.
At the moment that the anterior mitral leaflet (AML) is closing, the chordae show a systolic anterior motion (arrow). In this patient the SAM was not caused by the AML. There was also no mitral insufficiency during angiocardiography.

moment it is not yet necessary that mitral regurgitation results: the line of closure of the mitral leaflets is far from the leaflet tips. Thus, the mitral ostium may be still closed at the moment that part of the anterior leaflet is sucked into the outflow tract (Fig. 5).

This conception also explains why the SAM is not specific for HCM with obstruction but can also be found in other conditions and even sometimes in the hearts of young, healthy people.

In general, measurements of wall thicknesses or internal diameters of cavities can be made directly from the 2-D image or from an M-mode recording if the sound beam crosses the structures perpendicularly and the direction of motion is known. If the spatial position of the sound beam is not known, most measurements will be too great from M-mode.

The same is the case for the thickness of the IVS. The recorded thickness on

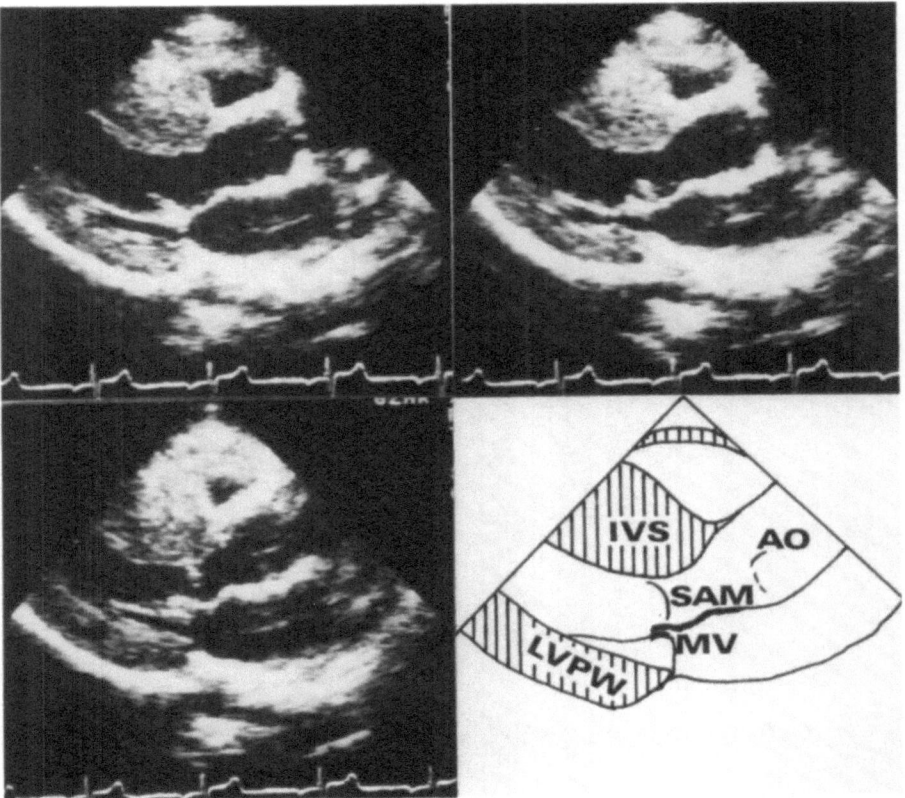

Figure 5. Long axis view of the heart of a patient with a high septal HCM with obstruction. All pictures have been made in early systole and the development of the SAM can be seen. From the picture on the bottom left it can be seen that the SAM is caused by the chordae and not by the still closed anterior mitral leaflet. For explanation see Figure 1.

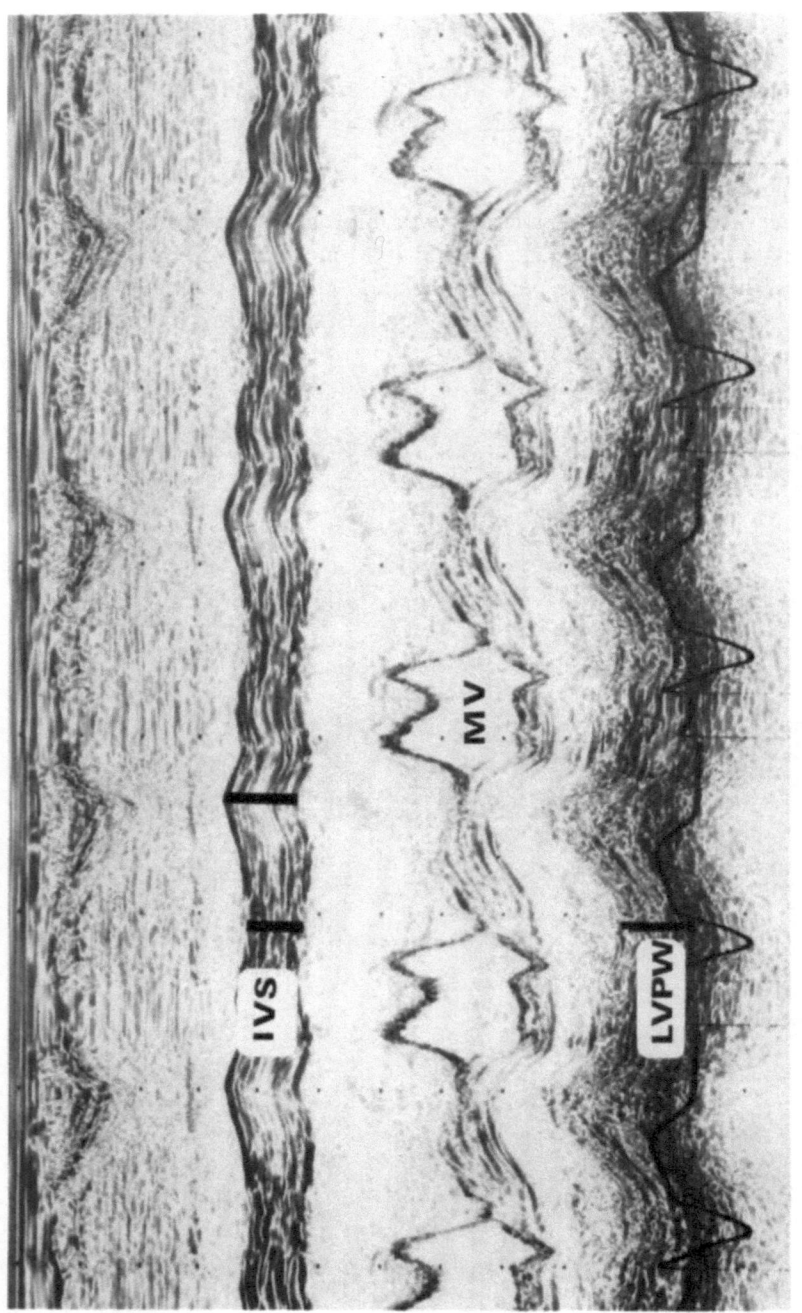

Figure 6. M-mode recording of the heart of a patient with a low septal-apical localization of HCM, assessed with 2-D echocardiography. The M-mode recording at the tip of the mitral valve (MV) shows the same thickness as the IVS and LVPW because the septal thickening was present in lower parts of the IVS. The difference between both is found in the nearly absent motion pattern of the IVS. Also the echo-density of the IVS is more than that of the LVPW. From the flutter on the anterior mitral leaflet it can also be concluded that this patient had aortic regurgitation as well.

M-mode not only depends on the angle between the IVS and the sound beam but also on the position of the whole ventricle and the localization of the thickened part of it. A mid or apical localization can result in a normal septal thickness on M-mode (Fig. 6).

If the ventricle is not crossed by the sound plane in the middle, the IVS and LVPW seem to be thicker than normal and the internal diameters of the ventricle smaller than the real dimensions (Fig. 7).

The motion of the various structures of the heart adds a new problem to this. It is not always known if a recorded motion represents a *passive* or an *active motion*. If a part of the heart cannot have an active motion as the aortic root, a passive motion will be recorded on M-mode, caused by a motion of the whole heart. The same is than the case for the most upper part of the IVS. We called this passive motion the *septal shift*. The M-mode recording of the muscular part of the IVS is not only influenced by this septal shift but also by the angle between the sound beam and the IVS. This can only be detected with 2-D echocardiography which makes the measurements of septal thickness and thickening rate with single crystal echocardiography in the past unreliable, including part of the conclusions made from these measurements.

In order to assess the diagnosis HCM a difference in thickness and thickening rate of a part of the ventricles has to be found.

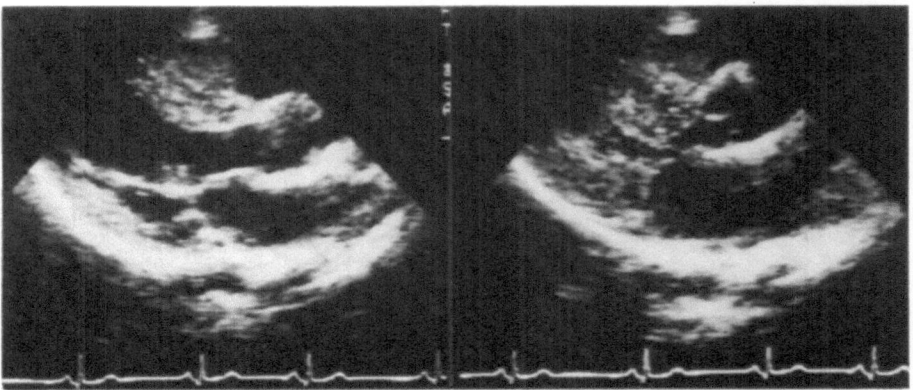

Figure 7. Long axis view of the heart of a patient with HCM. The basal part of the IVS is thickened. The LVPW has a normal thickness during diastole (left). At the end of systole (right) the total left ventricle has moved with its mid-portion out of the sound plane. As a consequence the IVS seems to have moved downward and the LVPW is much more thickened than is possible. An M-mode recording through the area below the mitral valve would suggest a good motion pattern of the IVS and an enormous thickening of the LVPW, leading to false measurements.

18

Figure 8 illustrates a few simplified problems that have to be recognized if an M-mode recording is made from a passively moving structure – without 'septal' thickening and without active excursion. Depending on the direction in which this 'dead' structure is moved or on the part of it that is hit by the sound plane, one can be able to record on M-mode a thinner IVS, a not existing systolic thickening or thinning and other untruthful findings. The examples only include a few very simplified problems.

In conclusion, for the diagnosis of HCM attention should be paid to the presence

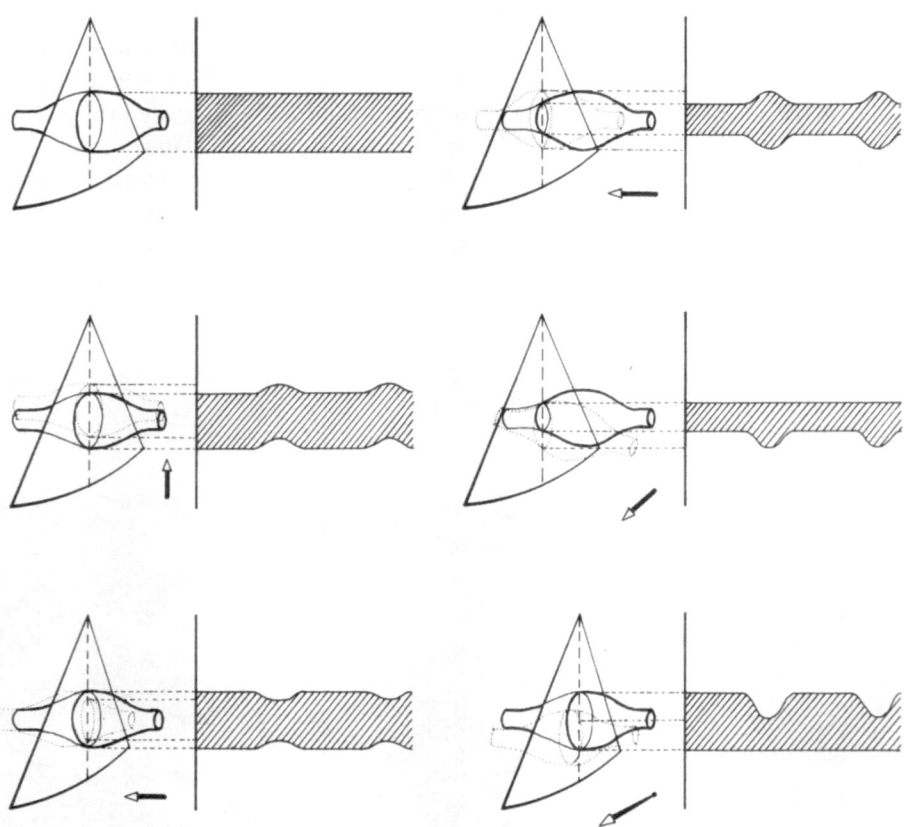

Figure 8. Schematic representation of the effect of a passively moving ovally shaped structure through a sound plane (triangle) on the M-mode recording (horizontal bars). Without a motion pattern a thickened 'IVS' without any motion will be recorded (top left). If the 'IVS' is only moved in upward direction (middle left), the same will be recorded on M-mode. A horizontal shift of the 'IVS' with a local thickening will result in a systolic thinning (bottom left), but depending on the part of the IVS that is crossed by the sound plane it can also result in a systolic thickening (upper right). An angulation downward and to the left can result in a one-sided pseudo thickening (middle right) and if a motion pattern toward the observer is added to this, a one-sided systolic thinning can be recorded. In reality, in all examples there is no thickening or thinning present from this 'IVS'.

of a local thickening of some part of the ventricles in combination with a diminished or lost thickening rate.

This can only be achieved by building up in mind a three-dimensional image of the heart composed from two-dimensional echocardiographic images, obtained from as many views as possible. The diagnosis can be supported with M-mode echocardiography with many restrictions.

References

1. Shah PM, Gramiak R, Kramer DH: Ultrasound localization of left ventricular outflow tract obstruction in hypertrophic cardiomyopathy. Circulation 40:3, 1969.
2. Popp RL, Harrison DC: Ultrasound in the diagnosis and evaluation of therapy of idiopathic hypertrophic subaortic stenosis. Circulation 40:905, 1969.
3. Abbasi AS, MacAlpin RN, Eber LM, Pearce ML: Echocardiographic diagnosis of idiopathic hypertrophic cardiomyopathy without outflow obstruction. Circulation 46:897, 1972.
4. Henry WL, Clark CE, Epstein SE: Asymmetric septal hypertrophy. Echocardiographic identification of the pathognomonic anatomic abnormality of IHSS. Circulation 47:225 1973.
5. Henry WL, Clark CE, Glancy DL, Epstein SE: Echocardiographic measurement of the left ventricular outflow gradient in idiopathic hypertrophic subaortic stenosis. N Engl J Med 288, 19:989, 1973.
6. Rossen RM, Goodman DJ, Ingham RE, Popp RL: Ventricular systolic septal thickening and excursion in idiopathic hypertrophic subaortic stenosis. N Eng J Med 291, 25:1317, 1974.
7. Tajik AJ, Giuliani ER: Echocardiographic observations in idiopathic subaortic stenosis. Mayo Clin Proc 49:89, 1974.
8. Cohen MV, Cooperman LB, Rosenblum R: Regional myocardial function in idiopathic hypertrophic subaortic stenosis. Circulation 52:842, 1975.
9. Henry WL, Clark CE, Griffith JM, Epstein SE: Mechanism of left ventricular outflow tract obstruction in patients with obstructive asymmetric septal hypertrophy (idiopathic subaortic stenosis). Am J Cardiol 35:337, 1975.
10. Cohen MV, Teichholz LE, Gorlin R: B-scan ultrasonography in idiopathic hypertrophic subaortic stenosis. Study of left ventricular outflow tract and mechanism of obstruction. Brit Heart J 38:595, 1976.
11. Chahine RA, Raizner AE, Ishimori T, Montero AC: Echocardiographic, haemodynamic, and angiographic correlations in hypertrophic cardiomyopathy. Brit Heart J 39:945, 1977.
12. Hamer JPM: Errors in echocardiographic measurements. M-mode versus two-dimensional registrations of the left heart. Abstracts 4th world congress on Ultrasonics in Medicine, Miyazaki, 1979, p 237.
13. DeMaria AN, Bommer W, Lee G, Mason DT: Value and limitations of two-dimensional echocardiography in assessment of cardiomyopathy. Am J Cardiol 46:1224, 1980.
14. Maron BJ, Gottdiener JS, Bonow RO, Epstein SE: Hypertrophic cardiomyopathy with unusual locations of left ventricular hypertrophy undetectable by M-mode echocardiography. Identification by wide-angle two-dimensional echocardiography. Circulation 63:409, 1981.
15. Maron BJ, Gottdiener JS, Bonow RO, Epstein SE: Patterns and significance of left ventricular hypertrophy in hypertrophic cardiomyopathy. A wide-angle, two-dimensial echocardiographic study of 125 patients. Am J Cardiol 48:418, 1981.
16. Maron BJ, Wolfson JK, Ciro É, Spirito P: Relation of electrocardiographic abnormalities and patterns of left ventricular hypertrophy identified by 2-dimensional echocardiography in patients with hypertrophic cardiomypathy. Am J Cardiol 51:189, 1983.
17. Shapiro LM, McKenna WJ: Distribution of left ventricular hypertrophy in hypertrophic cardiomyopathy: a two-dimensional echocardiographic study. JACC 2:437, 1983.

3. Arrhythmias in hypertrophic cardiomyopathy: prognostic significance and clinical relevance

J.W. VIERSMA, D.J. VAN VELDHUISEN, J.P.M. HAMER,
D.S. POSTMA and E. VAN DER WALL

Abstract. Eighty patients with hypertrophic cardiomyopathy were studied for the presence of ventricular and supraventricular arrhythmias by 24-hr ambulatory electrocardiography. Ventricular tachycardia was present in 18% of the recordings but was not correlated with any of the other manifestations of the disease and it was always asymptomatic. Supraventricular tachycardia, present in 13% of the recordings, was more often present in patients with palpitations.

Sixty-seven patients entered a follow-up study for the presence and prognostic significance of cardiac arrhythmias without any systematical intervention with anti-arrhythmic drugs. These patients were followed for a mean period of 4.9 years (1–8 years). The mean age of the patients was 36.7 years. During follow-up five patients died (7.5%), two of sudden death (3.0%). The mortality in this group of 67 patients with ventricular tachycardia at follow-up was 15.4% (two of 13), from which 7.7% (or one of 13) sudden death. This mortality is low in comparison to other follow-up trials.

Although the percentage of patients with ventricular tachycardia at the first 24-hr ambulatory ECG is approximately equal to the percentage at the last recording, there is a considerable individual variation: fifty percent of patients with ventricular tachycardia showed this arrhythmia only on one of these two recordings.

Introduction

Hypertrophic cardiomyopathy is a slowly progressive disorder of the heart muscle with a high incidence of sudden death often without warning symptoms. Sudden death is the main cause of death at young age. Ventricular arrhythmias are frequently found in hypertrophic cardiomyopathy. Like in coronary artery disease there have been many attempts to link the presence of ventricular arrhythmias with the occurrence of sudden death. The latter, however, is nearly always unexpected and a direct causal relation between a cardiac arrhythmia and sudden death is difficult to prove. Predictive value of ventricular arrhythmias for sudden death has been shown in several studies [1, 2]. Although some authors have also shown a relation between sudden death and other risk indicators in patients with hypertrophic cardiomyopathy like family history, young age and syncopal attacks [3–6], no study showed a direct prognostic relation of any invasive or non-invasive parameter in hypertrophic cardiomyopathy with sudden cardiac death [7, 8]. This relation was not found between cardiac arrhythmias and morphological criteria or symptoms either.

In the present study we used 24-hr ambulatory electrocardiography (DECG) to detect the frequency and types of arrhythmias in patients with hypertrophic cardiomyopathy. We investigated a possible prognostic significance of these arrhythmias in a prospective follow-up and looked for a relation of the arrhythmias with other manifestations of hypertrophic cardiomyopathy.

Patients and methods

Eighty patients with the diagnosis hypertrophic cardiomyopathy were studied; they entered the study without any other criterion for selection! The diagnosis was based upon echocardiographic data of asymmetrical septal hypertrophy and the a-wave of the apex cardiogram. Cardiac catheterization and cineangiography was performed in 90% of the patients.

Sixty-seven patients were first studied with a 24-hr ambulatory electrocardiogram (DECG) in the period 1976–1982. Many of these patients had been followed for a number of years in our out-patient clinic before the study started. Surgical therapy for hypertrophic cardiomyopathy, e.g. septal myotomy or myectomy, was performed in eight patients a long time before the study started; in five of them before 1970, more than 6 years before entry to the study.

Thirteen patients, however, were studied for the first time in 1983 or 1984 and they were not considered in the follow-up. Of the 67 patients who were studied by 24-hr DECG, 42 were males (63%) and 25 were females (37%); ages ranged from 13–63 years, with a mean age of 36.7 years at entry. Children below the age of thirteen were not included in this follow-up because these patients were seen in the department of pediatric cardiology.

Patients were followed until 1983–1984 for 1–8 years or a total of 293 patients-years, with a mean follow-up time of 4.9 years. A second 24-hr DECG was recorded at the end of this period in 58 patients. Five patients died during follow-up and four patients, although alive, were out of the catchment area. DECG recordings were performed on a Avionics 445 recorder and analyzed by personal supervision on a Avionics 680 analyzer. Ventricular arrhythmias were classified according to Ryan, Lown et al. [9]:

grade 0: no VPB
grade I: occasional VPBs, up to a maximum of 30 in any of the recorded hours
grade II: more than 30 VPBs in any hour recorded
grade III: multiform VPBs
grade IVa: two consecutive VPBs
grade IVB: ventricular tachycardia (three or more VPBs in succession)

During the recording patients stayed at home and were kept on their regularly used medication. Medical treatment was based on symptoms and consisted, at time of the follow-up, of 38 of 71 patients (54%) on beta blocking agents. Thirty one were on a daily dose of less than 160 mg propranolol or an equivalent dose of another beta blocker. Seven patients used a dose of propranolol or equivalent of 160 mg per day or more up to a maximum dose of 320 mg per day.

Verapamil was used in 11% of the patients. Class I anti-arrhythmic drugs (quinidine or disopyramide) were used in 11% of the patients. Amiodarone was used at the time of follow-up by 8% of the patients. There was no systematical treatment for ventricular arrhythmias. Twenty-three percent of the patients used no medical therapy during the follow-up registration.

When a patients experienced palpitations during the 24-hr ambulatory electrocardiography, as was frequently present in many patients, they could mark the recording with a so-called 'event-button'. In this way we were able to trace a possible correlation between symptoms and cardiac arrhythmias.

Results

At the first recording ventricular tachycardia was present in 19.4% and in the second study in 17.2% of the patients. This percentage is fairly well in agreement with the observations of other authors in patients with hypertrophic cardiomyopathy [8, 10, 11–13] but it is much higher than the occurrence of ventricular tachycardia in normal individuals of the same age group [14], as is shown in Table 1.

Supraventricular tachycardia was present at entry in seven out of 67 patients (10.4%) and at the second recording in eight out of 58 patients (14%). Atrial fibrillation was present at entry in 2 patients and at the follow-up in three patients.

Ventricular tachycardia was present in a non-sustained form (Fig. 1) but it was

Table 1. (Ventricular arrhythmias according to the Ryan and Lown classification. Comparison with other studies and with normal individuals)

	Present series Entry	Follow-up		McKenna [10]	Canedo [11]	Savage [8]	Bjarnason [12]	Bourmayan [13]	Manger Cats [14] Normals	
n	67	58		30	33	100	22	21	300	
0	26.9 %	15.5	%						23.3	%
I	25.4 %	22.4	%						38.7	%
II	6.0 %	1.7	%						2.7	%
III	13.4 %	20.7	%						21.7	%
IV[a]	9.0 %	22.4	%						12.7	%
IV[b]	19.4 %	17.2	%	17%	15%	19%	14%	14%	1.7	%

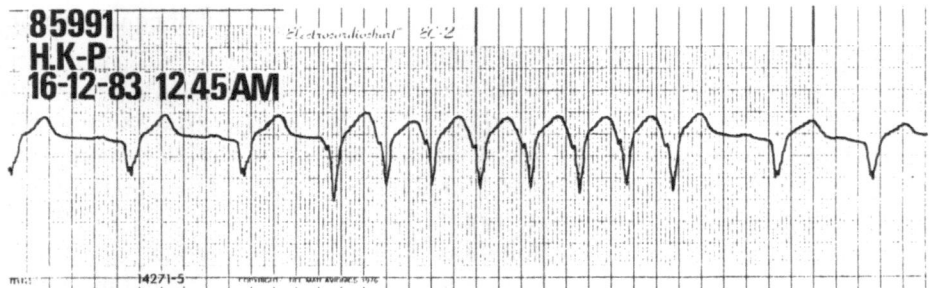

Figure 1. Non-sustained ventricular tachycardia, unobserved by the patient.

always unobserved by the patients. Many patients on the other hand experienced palpitations even during the same recording, but not at the moment of ventricular tachycardia. When asked by standardized question form, palpitations were mentioned by 53% of the patients and there was no correlation at all with the presence of ventricular tachycardia. So, thusfar we could not find any correlation between the presence of ventricular tachycardia and the presence of symptomes like syncope (10%), angina pectoris (46%) or dizziness (46%).

In patients with supraventricular tachycardia palpitations were present significantly more often, that is in 15 of 18 recordings of patients with supraventricular tachycardia (Fig. 2).

Although the number of patients with ventricular tachycardia was quite comparable between the beginning and the end of the study, the individual variability was large (Fig. 3). Of 12 patients who had ventricular tachycardia at entry to the study, only five (42%) showed this arrhythmia during follow-up; two patients had died, one of sudden death. Five patients showed a lesser degree of ventricular arrhythmia at follow-up. Of the 10 patients with ventricular tachycardia during the second study, five had a lesser degree of arrhythmia at entry to the study.

In the first study, coupled beats were only present in 3/13 = 23% of those who show coupled beats at follow-up. In most instances however, a 24-hr DECG showed, when the arrhythmia was present, several pairs of VPBs, while with

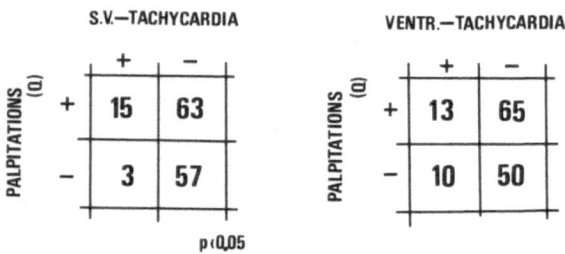

Figure 2. Relation between palpitations and the presence of supraventricular tachycardia and relation between palpitations and the presence of ventricular tachycardia. There is only a positive relation between palpitations and supraventricular tachycardia. The numbers represent the number of 24–hr ambulatory ECG recordings.

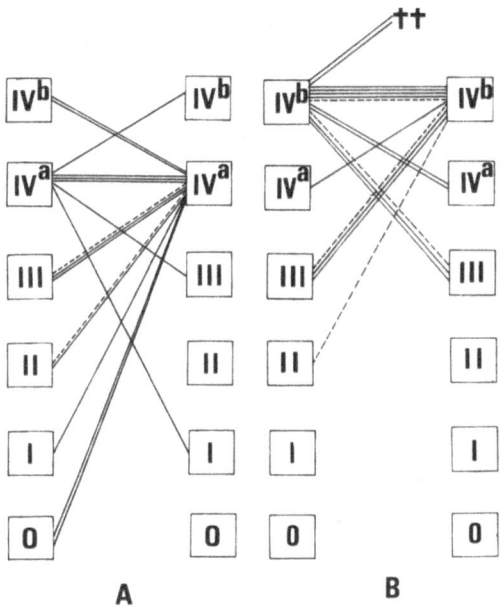

Figure 3. Variability of high grade ventricular arrhythmias. Every patient is represented by a line. Broken lines indicate the addition of anti–arrhytmic drugs during follow–up. The left–hand columns represent the data at entry and the right–hand columns represent the data at follow–up. A: patients with paired VPBs on one or both of the recordings; B: patients with ventricular tachycardia on one or both of the recordings.

ventricular tachycardia, when present, half of them occurred only once during a recording. The length of the recording may therefore be of considerable influence on this variability in ventricular tachycardia.

In supraventricular tachycardia the variability was even larger, as is shown in Figure 4. Only in one patient supraventricular tachycardia was present in both instances. Several manifestations of hypertrophic cardiomyopathy as can be shown with non-invasive diagnostic techniques were tested and a possible correlation with the degree of ventricular arrhythmia was looked for. In an earlier study in our department [15] the height of the a-wave of the apex cardiogram, which is an expression of the compliance of the left ventricle, seemed to have some predictive value for ventricular tachycardia. Figure 5 shows that we could not prove a correlation between the a-wave heigth and the class of ventricular arrhythmias in these patients. There was no correlation either with the septum thickness, as measured by sector echocardiography, nor with the ratio between septum and left ventricular free wall diameter. Also there was no predictive value for any of the electrocardiographic criteria like the voltage ($S_{V1} + R_{V5}$ or R_{V6}), pseudo-infarction patterns or the length of the QT-interval.

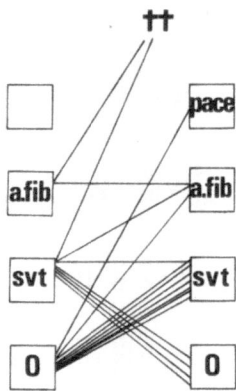

Figure 4. Variability in supraventricular arrhythmias. Every patient is represented by a line; pace = artificial pacemaker rhythm; a.fib = atrial fibrillation; svt = supraventricular tachycardia; 0 = none of the above–mentioned supraventricular arrhythmias.

Follow-up and prognosis

During the follow-up period with a mean of 4.9 years (range 1–8 years) five patients died, two of sudden death. The other three patients died of non-cardiac causes. This accounts for a total death rate of 3.0%. Of the 13 patients with ventricular tachycardia at the first 24-hr DECG the rate of sudden death was 1/13 (7.7%) and the total death rate was 2/13 (15.4%).

The annual rate of sudden death of patients with ventricular tachycardia in our study is below 2% per year, which is low compared to other studies. Maron et al. [2] found an annual mortality rate for sudden death in patients with ventricular tachycardia of 8.9% and McKenna [16] found an even higher percentage.

Discussion

Sudden death is often seen in the course of hypertrophic cardiomyopathy. The true mechanism is not exactly known but many authors speculate that it is arrhythmic in origin [1, 2, 6]. The frequent occurrence of ventricular tachycardia in hypertrophic cardiomyopathy on long–term ECG registrations make it likely to suggest not just a predictive value – a risk indicator – as has been shown in several studies, but also a causal relationship.

Sudden death encountered in retrospective casualties in hypertrophic cardio-myopathy was more frequently seen in patients of the younger age groups. Maron [6] showed that the age of the majority of patients with sudden death was

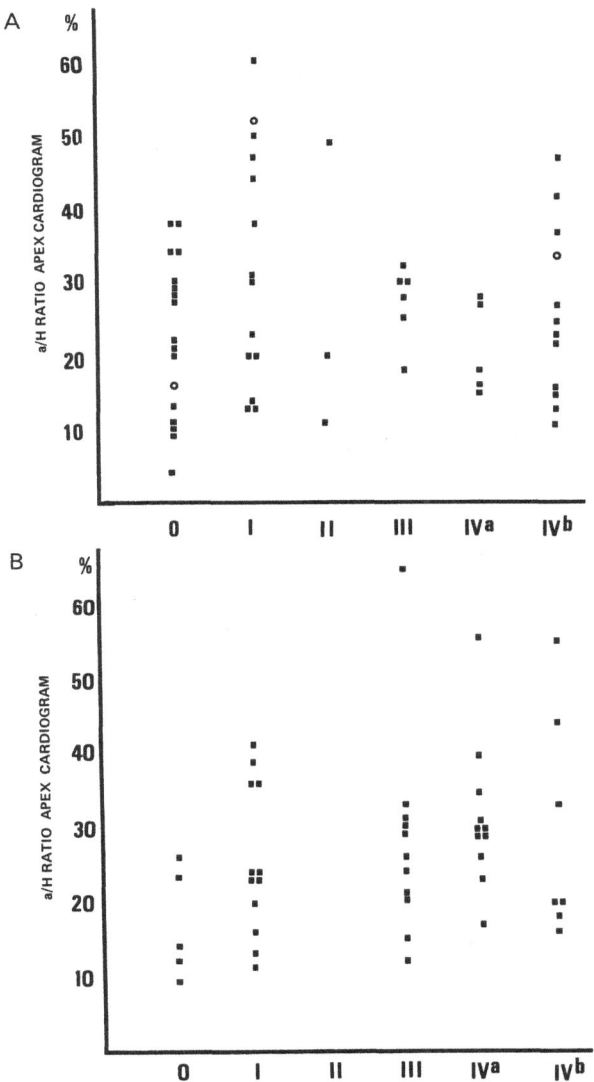

Figure 5. Relation between a–wave height of the apexcardiogram and the degree of ventricular arrhythmias (Lown classification) at entry (A) and at follow–up (B). Open symbols represent patients who died during the follow–up.

below 30 years. In our own department (Fig. 6) sudden death was also more common in patients below 30 as well, again looked at in retrospective manner.

In this prospective study, the rate of sudden death was low, despite an equal number of patients with ventricular tachycardia. The age of our patients was also comparable to the other studies with a mean age of 36.7 years, while in the study of Maron et al. [2] this was 38 years and a mean age of 39 years in the study of McKenna et al [1].

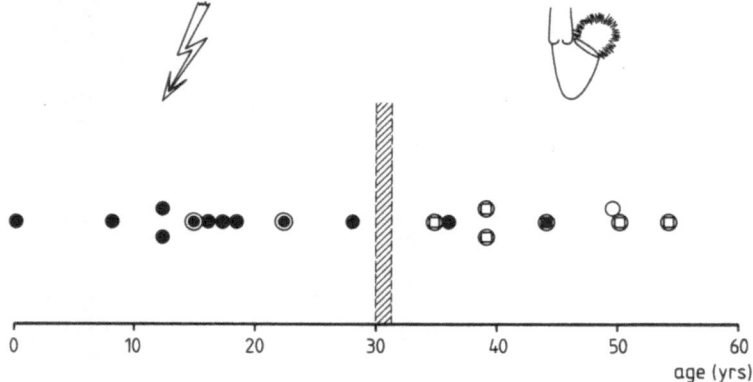

Figure 6. Causes of death in 18 patients with HCM in a retrospective study (unpublished data). Below the age of 30 years, sudden 'electrical' death predominates, not completely prevented by beta blocking agents. Beyond the age of 30 years 'mechanical' death, frequently induced by atrial fibrillation, prevails.
● = sudden death; □ = atrial fibrillation; ■ = heart failure; ○ = non-cardiac; encircled symbols indicate patients on beta blocking therapy.

Looking at the age of patients in the different classes of arrhythmia, like in Figure 7, we could not find an inverse relation of the degree of the ventricular arrhythmias and age; on the contrary, the mean age in the patients with ventricular tachycardia seems to be at least as high as the mean age of all patients. If ventricular tachycardia is a forerunner of sudden death, one might expect, in view of the retrospective data, ventricular tachycardia more often in younger

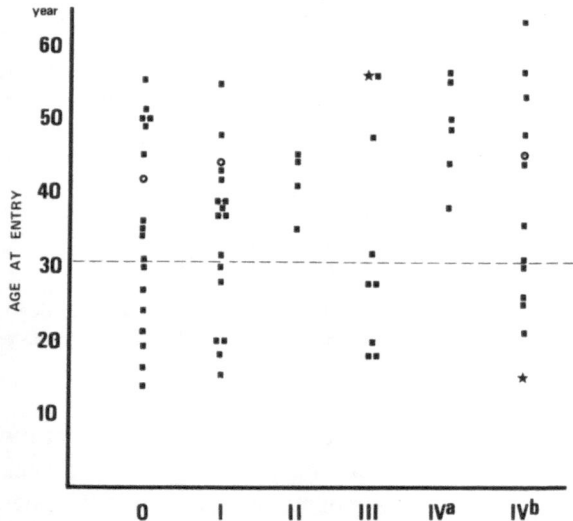

Figure 7. Relation of age of patients with hypertrophic cardiomyopathy and the degree of ventricular arrhythmias (Lown classification). ■ = alive at follow-up; ○ died (non-cardiac cause); ★ = sudden death during follow-up.

patients which however is not found in our data. Another factor to be considered as explanation for the low mortality in our patients may be the long period of follow-up in our out-patient clinic after the diagnosis was made, but before the patients entered the study with the first 24-hr DECG. Patients with a rapidly progressive deterioration of the disease may possibly have died shortly after the diagnosis was made and can have been missed by natural selection in the period before the first analysis of arrhythmias. The period between establishment of the diagnosis and entrance to this study is however comparable to the one in other studies mentioned.

The predictive value of ventricular tachycardia for sudden death in our patients was lower than of comparable groups of patients in the literature [1, 2].

Treatment

The patients in the present study were not systematically treated for ventricular arrhythmias.

Maron [2] states that the mortality of patients with hypertrophic cardiomyopathy who show ventricular tachycardia on ambulatory electrocardiograms is high enough to warrant therapeutic intervention. However, no evidence is available that anti-arrhythmic therapy will prevent sudden death in these patients, even when ventricular tachycardias are abolished.

Frank [17] advocates aggressive search for and treatment of so-called 'potentially lethal arrhythmias'. Besides ventricular tachycardia this author considers paired ventricular ectopic beats and supraventricular tachycardias potentially lethal as well. He uses beta blocking drugs in a high dose, until the resting standing heart rate is approximately 60 beats per minute and calls this 'complete beta blockade'. Thus treated the mean dose of propranolol is about 480 mg daily, which is high above the generally used dosages, and much higher than dosages we have used. His study showed that even with these dosages the majority of paired beats and ventricular tachycardias were not suppressed, and therefore class I anti-arrhythmic drugs were added. Most effective in his experience, in combination with high doses of propranolol, were quinidine and disopyramide. Finally the mortality per year in this study is low: 0.3% per year for sudden death in 50 patients. However, the age of the patients in this study was relatively high with a mean of 49.4 years, which could be an important factor to explain the low incidence of sudden death. McKenna showed that verapamil [1] even in high dosages given to suppress symptoms, will not suppress ventricular tachycardia. Amiodarone [18] did effectively reduce ventricular tachycardia in 10 of 13 patients, but was even more effective in abolition of supraventricular arrhythmias. McKenna finds only little effect of the use of beta-blockers in the suppression of ventricular tachycardia.

In our study much lower dosages of beta blockers were used. In Figure 8 the

30

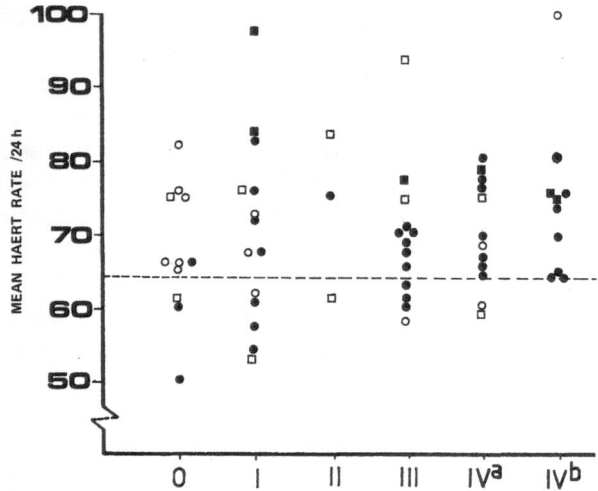

Figure 8. Relation between mean heart rate during the 24–hr registration and the degree of ventricular arrhythmias (Lown classification). Symbols represent the main cardiac drug regimen at the time of registration during the follow–up. ● = beta blocking agent; □ = verapamil; ■ = anti–arrhythmia drug; ○ = none.

mean heart rate during the 24–hr DECG was compared of all individual patients. Again the patients were arranged according to the class of ventricular arrhythmias. Despite treatment with beta blockers the daily mean heart rate was above 64/min in patients with ventricular tachycardia. The difference with lower classes of ventricular arrhythmias was however non–significant.

Conclusion

Our study does not support the unfavourable prognosis for patients with HCM who are identified to have ventricular tachycardia or a lower degree of ventricular arrhythmias. Therefore our study does not support the view that aggressive treatment of ventricular tachycardia in these patients is mandatory. These non-sustained ventricular tachycardias are symptomless, are present with an individual variability in 24–hr DECG recordings, and are present to the same extent in the older age groups, where death is often due to pump failure in contrast with the young age groups where sudden death predominates.

References

1. McKenna WJ, England D, Doi YL, Deanfield JE, Oakley C, Goodwin JF: Arrhythima in HCM. I. Influence on prognosis. Br Heart J, 46: 168–172, 1981.

2. Maron BJ, Savage DD, Wolfson JK, Epstein SE: Prognostic significance of 24 hour ambulatory ECG monitoring in patients with HCM. A prospective study. Am J Cardiol 48: 252 – 257, 1981.
3. Hardarson T, de la Calzada CS, Curiel R, Goodwin JF: Prognosis and mortality of HOCM. Lancet 11: 1462 – 1469, 1973.
4. McKenna WJ, Deanfield J, Faruqui D, England D, Oackley C, Goodwin JF: Prognosis in HCM, Role of age and clinical, electrocardiographic and hemodynamic features. Am J Cardiol 47: 532 – 538, 1981.
5. Maron BJ, Lipson LC, Roberts WC, Savage DD, Epstein SE: 'Malignant' hypertrophic cardiomyopathy: identification of a subgroup of families with unusually frequent premature death. Am J Cardiol. 41: 1133 – 1140, 1978.
6. Maron BJ, Roberts WC, Epstein SE: Sudden death in hypertrophic cardiomyopathy: a profile of 78 patients. Circulation 65: 1388 – 1394, 1982.
7. Doi Y, McKenna WJ, Chetty S, Oakley C, Goodwin JF: Prediction of mortality and serious ventricular arrhythmia in hypertrophic cardiomyopathy. Brit Heart J 44: 150 – 157, 1980.
8. Savage DD, Seides SF, Maron BJ, Myers DJ, Epstein SE: Prevalence of arrhythmias during 24–hour electrocardiographic monitoring and exercise testing in patients with obstructive and non–obstructive hypertrophic cardiomyopathy. Circulation 59: 860 – 875, 1979.
9. Ryan M, Lown B, Horn H: Ventricular ectopic activity in patients with coronary heart disease. N. Engl J Med 292: 224 – 229, 1975.
10. McKenna WJ, Chetty S, Oakley C, Goodwin JF: Arrhythmia in hypertrophic cardiomyopathy: exercise and 48 hour ambulatory electrocardiographic assessment with and without beta adrenergic blocking therapy. Am J Cardiol 45: 1 – 5, 1980.
11. Canedo MJ, Frank MJ, Abdulla AM: Rhythm disturbances in hypertrophic cardiomyopathy: prevalence, relation to symptoms and management. Am J Cardiol 45: 848 – 855, 1980.
12. Bjarnason I, Hardarson T, Johnsson S: Cardiac arrhythmias in hypertrophic cardiomyopathy. Brit Heart J 48: 198 – 203, 1982.
13. Bourmayan C, Nouhad M, Fournier C, Bouajina A, Desnos M, Gay J, Gerbaux A: Arythmies ventriculaires de la myocardiopathie hypertrophique obstructive. La Presse Medicale 12: 2089 – 2092, 1983.
14. Manger Cats V, Durrer D: Prevalence of cardiac arrhythmias in the normal active population. In: Roeland J, Hugenholt PG (ed), Long–term Ambulatory Electrocardiography. Martinus Nijhoff, The Hague, 1982.
15. Viersma JW, van der Wall E: Hypertrophische cardiomyopathie en ritmestoornissen bij 24–uurs dynamische electrocardiografie. Ned T Geneesk. 125: 2116, 1981.
16. McKenna WJ: Arrhythmias in hypertrophic cardiomyopathy. Eur Heart J 4 (suppl F): 225 – 234, 1983.
17. Frank MJ, Stefadouros MA, Watkins LO, Prisant LM, Abdulla AM: Rhythm disturbances in hypertrophic cardiomyopathies: relationship to symptoms and the effect of 'complete' beta blockade. Eur Heart J (suppl F): 235 – 243, 1983.
18. McKenna WJ, Harris L, Perez G, Krikler DM, Oakley C, Goodwin JF: Arrhythmias in hypertrophic cardiomyopathy II. Comparison of amiodarone and verapamil in treatment. Brit Heart J 46: 173 – 178, 1981.

4. Cardiomyopathies: evaluation with radionuclide techniques

E.E. VAN DER WALL

Introduction

In recent years radioactive tracers have been used more extensively in the care of patients with coronary artery disease (CAD), valvular lesions, intracardiac shunts and cardiomyopathies. It has been predicted that radionuclide techniques will achieve a role in cardiology equal in importance to electrocardiography, echocardiography and cardiac catheterization.

Several factors have contributed to the progress in nuclear cardiology. The first is the development of gamma scintillation cameras with better spatial resolution. The second is the availability of medically suitable radiopharmaceuticals which will selectively localize in the normal or injured myocardium. The third involves minicomputers and microprocessors which are nowadays fast, powerful and compact and allow the processing and storing of large volumes of data at a relatively low cost. Fourth, since radionuclide studies are non-invasive, they can easily be repeated and interventions can be studied at short term. At last, radionuclide studies provide information of cardiac function which can not be given with other diagnostic techniques. For example, recent research with cyclotron-produced radioisotopes, such as free fatty acids (FFA) labeled with carbon-11 or iodine-123, indicates that is possible to study regional myocardial metabolism and to differentiate diseases characterized by a decreased supply of blood from those characterized by an increased demand of substrate. Not only in CAD, but also in idiopathic cardiomyopathy, such studies may be valuable to improve our understanding of disease processes.

In this review, attention will be focused on the value of radionuclide techniques for the detection of cardiomyopathies, in particular hypertrophic cardiomyopathy. Before entering these issues, the currently available cardiovascular nuclear medicine procedures will be discussed. Broadly speaking, the fall into two major categories: those concerned with the heart as a *muscle* and those concerned with the heart as a *pump*.

Cardiac instrumentation

The function of the gammacamera is to convert radioactivity into a pictorial representation. The current detection system consists of a collimator, one or more crystals, photomultiplier tubes and an electronic circuit. The collimator is a device made of lead, which absorbs gamma rays (photons) traveling in a direction other than a straight line from the heart. The photons interact with the crystal(s) to produce visual light. The produced scintillations are converted to an electronic signal by photomultiplier tubes. The electronic signals are computed as X,Y signals and visualized on an oscilloscope on the camera console as well as sent to a computer for subsequent data analysis.

The gammacamera is a stationary or mobile system, with a field of view from 18 to 40 cm diameter, positioned over the chest cage. One version of this, the single-probe detector or nuclear stethoscope, has a small field of view of about 5 cm, and is also rapidly gaining acceptance for monitoring of left ventricular function. The probe offers the advantage of true portability, decreased cost and enhanced detector sensitivity. However, only temporal information can be obtained (beat-to-beat analysis) but no spatial information is provided (non-imaging probe).

Radiopharmaceuticals

Radionuclides have three main characteristics: (1) type of emission i.e. radiation of alpha, beta, gamma or positron (i.e. beta-plus) rays, (2) level of energy – expressed in kiloelectronVolt (keV) –, and (3) physical and biological half-life. The ideal radionuclide for conventional cardiac evaluation should have the following properties: (1) a pure gamma emitting tracer with a photon energy of 100–200 keV, (2) a physical half-life of several hours to permit serial measurements over a short time period, (3) no pharmacologic effects which might affect physiological conditions, and (4) wide availability and low cost. So far, no currently used cardiac imaging agent meets all these requirements.

Regional myocardial blood flow

The most widely used tracer for the study of heart muscle is the radioisotope thallium-201 (half-life 72 hr, gamma emission 80 keV). After intravenous administration of 1.5–2 milliCuries (mCi), the initial distribution of thallium is related to the blood flow in the myocardium. In normal persons, between 85% and 90% of the arterial concentration is extracted by ventricular muscle in a single passage. Since coronary blood flow is 4–5% of the cardiac output, it follows that about 3% of the injected amount will be taken up by the healthy myocardium. Decreased coronary blood flow and/or reduced cellular extraction results in the appearance of a decrease in thallium concentration i.e. cold spots on gammacamera images.

Abnormalities are classified as regional or diffuse, as for example in CAD or congestive cardiomyopathy (CCM) respectively. While it is clear that CAD is associated with the appearance of clear regional defects, a thin-walled dilated ventricle in which the thallium-201 is mostly uniformly distributed, is more likely to be non-coronary. Occasionally, three-vessel disease may result in a uniform distribution of activity, but in such patients the ventricle is usually hypertrophied as indicated by the thickness of the ventricular walls on the thallium images. Although useful information can be obtained from thallium images in the acute stage of myocardial infarction i.e. the site and size of the infarction, the most common indication is the detection of suspected CAD during exercise thallium scintigraphy. The patients are usually exercised on a treadmill with an intravenous line inserted into a dorsal hand vein (fig. 1). A 12-lead electrocardiogram is obtained every 3 min and patients exercise until the appearance of symptoms (angina or fatique). The patients are injected with 1.5–2.0 mCi thallium-201 intravenously at maximum exercise and asked to continue the exercise for 30 sec during which time the thallium is effectively taken up by the heart muscle. Imaging starts preferably within 5 min after termination of the exercise with the use of a standard gammacamera interfaced with a nuclear medicine computer. We employ a low-energy all-purpose collimator with a 20% window around the 80 keV gammaline of thallium-201. Images of 6–8 min duration each are collected in the anterior, 45-degree and 70-degree left anterior oblique (LAO) positions (300.000 counts per image). The 3 projections are collected again 3–4 hr after the initial series of images without the need for an additional thallium injection. These late images are called delayed or redistribution images.

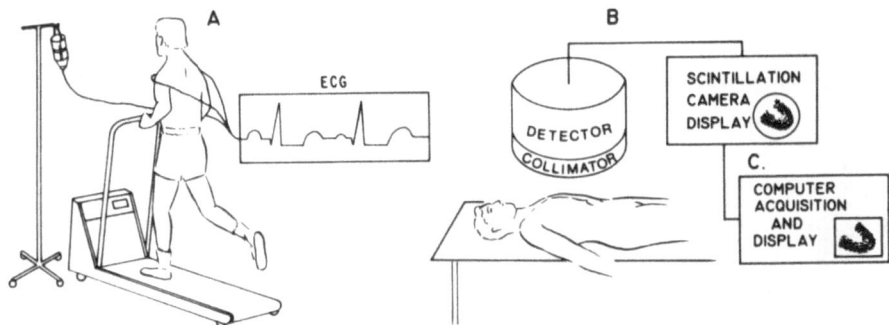

Figure 1. A. Exercise protocol for thallium scintigraphy. Patients are exercised according to Bruce protocol until the appearance of symptoms (angina, fatigue). At maximal exercise 2 mCi thallium is intravenously administered. B. Thereafter multiple view scintigraphic imaging takes place and 4–6 hr later redistribution images are performed. (Adapted from DS Berman and DT Mason, Clinical Nuclear Cardiology, Grune & Stratton, 1982).

Image interpretation

Figure 2 schematically demonstrates the three left ventricular views and the division of each projection into 3 segments. The 40- or 45-degree LAO view is often considered as the most important position, since this view provides the most optimal insight in the distribution of the 3 major coronary arteries. Adequate interpretation is achieved by visual comparison of the delayed and the exercise images. When both series of images are normal, it is very unlikely that the patient has CAD. However, in patients with serious CAD transient defects can be observed (Fig. 3). A transient defect is defined as a defect in at least one segment on the exercise image associated with a normalization of thallium activity on the delayed image. This finding denotes reversible ischemia and is mostly consistent with a hemodynamically significant stenosis in the coronary artery that supplies the segment. A persistent defect is defined as a defect on both the initial and the delayed images. Such a defect is thought to represent myocardial scar due to old infarction. Until now, it has been demonstrated that thallium exercise scintigraphy is superior to exercise electrocardiography for the detection of patients with CAD. Both sensitivity and specificity are significantly higher for exercise thallium imaging [1].

Assessment of morphology

Apart from detection of CAD by the observation of regional defects, the thallium image can provide information of the configuration and size of the left ventricle. This information is useful for the appropriate determination of the various forms of cardiomyopathies. A thick-walled septum will very likely correspond with a hypertrophic cardiomyopathy, while a thin-walled left ventricle associated with a large cavity mostly goes along with a dilated cardiomyopathy.

In normal circumstances, the right ventricle will not be visualized due to relatively less muscle mass and diminished blood supply compared to the left

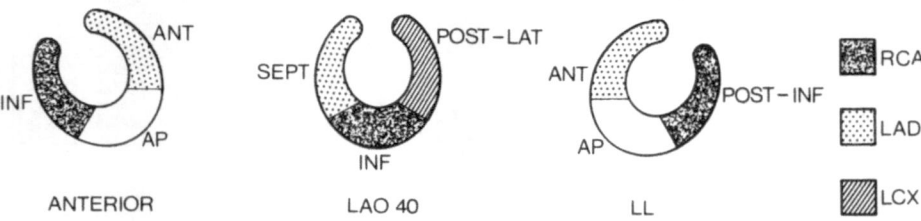

Figure 2. Schematic illustration of the myocardial segments analyzed on the thallium-201 images and the corresponding vascular beds. RCA = right coronary artery; LAD = left anterior descending coronary artery; LCX = left circumflex coronary artery; INF = inferior; AP = apical; ANT = anterior; SEPT = septal; POST = posterior; LAT = lateral; LAO 40 = 40-degree left anterior oblique; LL = left lateral.

ventricle. However, under exercise conditions or with right ventricular hypertrophy the right ventricle may be observed on the thallium image.

Cardiac metabolism

Cardiac disease is at present most frequently diagnosed and treated in its final stage i.e. when structural or anatomical derangements have already occurred. However, disease begins at the biochemical level and therapies are designed to terminate or reverse abnormal biochemical processes, restore delivery of biochemical nutrients or supplement depleted ones. Any technique that provides biochemically specific information about the myocardium could play a vital role in the early diagnosis and management of human cardiac disease. This holds in particular for cardiomyopathies, since classification of primary cardiomyopathies is currently based on anatomic and functional abnormalities regardless of the underlying etiology. Biochemical studies will enhance our understanding of these disorders as well as aid in the development of effective treatment.

Although the interest for metabolism of the human heart dates from many years ago, it is only recently that radiolabeled FFA can be applied for non-invasive metabolic studies of the myocardium.

FFA are preferred substrates for the normal myocardium and account for 70–80% of the energy production by the heart. In myocardial ischemia, there is an inhibition of FFA uptake in the myocardium, probably as a result of diminished coronary blood flow but also because of a shift to carbohydrate metabolism. FFA have been labeled with isotopes like carbon-11 (C-11) and iodine-123 (I-123). Since C-11 is a positron-emitting radioisotope, special tomographic devices (positron cameras) are needed, which strongly limit a wide applicability of C-11-labeled fatty acids. Conversely, I-123 is an excellent radioisotope for gam-

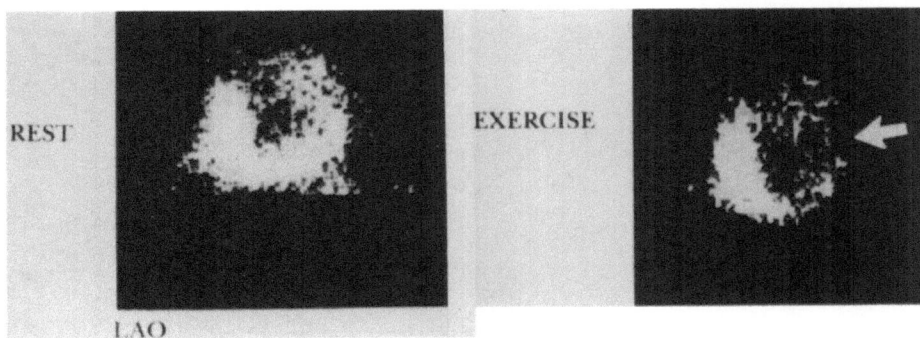

Figure 3. Exercise and redistribution (rest) thallium images in a patient with angina pectoris. After exercise, a prominent defect is seen in the posterolateral wall, while the distribution image 4 hr after thallium injection is normal. Coronary arteriography showed a significant lesion in the left circumflex coronary artery. LAO = left anterior oblique.

ma camera imaging (gamma energy 159 keV, half-life 13.3 hr). Initial results with FFA imaging I-123 labeled to hexadecanoic acid and to heptadecanoic acid) demonstrated that images are comparable to those obtained with thallium-201. Moreover, it has been shown that the metabolic turnover of FFA can be studied by the measurement of clearance rates from regional myocardium (Fig. 4). In clinical studies it has been reported that significantly different clearance rates were measured between normally perfused, transient ischemic and acutely infarcted regions. With reference to clearance rates determined from normal regions (half-time values of about 25 min), we observed increased values in ischemic regions and decreased values in infarcted regions (Fig. 5) [2, 3]. These findings suggest a slow metabolic turnover of I-123-FFA in reversibly injured myocardium and a fast turnover in irreversible ischemic myocardium. In this way, the use of I-123-FFA may rapidly assess the nature of myocardial ischemia. As for cardiomyopathies, it has been shown that the determination of clearance rates in patients with CCM could be valuable. Twenty patients with CCM showed inhomogeneous tracer distribution and slow clearance rates suggesting altered FFA metabolism in diseased myocardial regions [4]. In an other study, 9 patients with CCM and 6 patients with hypertrophic cardiomyopathy (HCM) were evaluated with I-123-heptadecanoic acid [5]. Compared to controls, clearance rates were reduced (i.e. slow metabolic turnover) in both groups of patients. The reduction in uptake was however more pronounced in patients with CCM than in those with HCM. The interpretation of diminished uptake and decreased clearance of FFA in patients with CCM and HCM is unclear at the present time. The

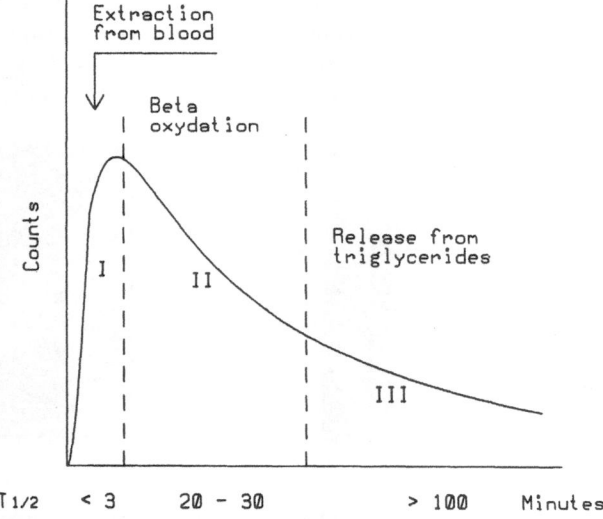

Figure 4. Schematic illustration of the characteristic time–activity curve of radiolabeled free fatty acids in the myocardium. Three distinct phases are recognized and expressed in minutes half-time ($T_{1/2}$).

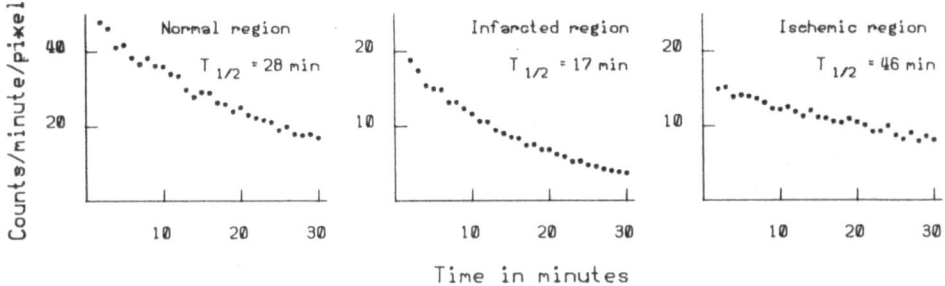

Figure 5. Time–activity curves derived from different myocardial regions. The curves are obtained after correction for free iodide. $T_{1/2}$ = myocardial half-time.

decrease in uptake may be caused by a disturbance of fatty acid transfer between extracellular binding sites on albumin whatever subcellular structures are involved. Regarding clearance, this may be reduced by a diminished demand for beta-oxidation or an alteration of the distibution of coenzyme A between the cytosol compartment and the intramitochondrial compartment. Also the carnitine shuttle across the mitochondrial membrane could be imcompetent, since it is supposed that the application of L-carnitine results in an improvement of fatty acid metabolism.

Whatever reason for the observed phenomenon, these data indicate the potential of I-123-FFA to provide insight in the pathophysiological and biochemical processes in patients with cardiomyopathies.

Cardiac function

Two techniques can be used for the assessment of cardiac function; (1) first-pass radionuclide angriography, and (2) multiple gated bloodpool scintigraphy. Usually for both methods technetium-99m (Tc-99m) is used as the imaging agent. The physical half-life of Tc-99m is 6 hr and its gamma energy 140 keV, ideally suited to current gammacameras.

First-pass radionuclide angiography

With the first-pass technique, 15 mCi Tc-99m pertechnetate is rapidly injected in an antecubital vein as a compact bolus. The scintillation data of the first pass through the central circulation are accumulated by a multi-crystal or single-crystal camera. Complete mixing of the bolus is assumed to have occurred by the time the radionuclide enters the left ventricle. As a result, changes in radioactivity during the ejection phase reflect proportional changes in chamber volume and are free of geometric assumptions. The efficacy of the first-pass method is dependent upon obtaining sufficiently high count rates to assume statistical accuracy. The multi-crystal camera provides a much higher count rate capacity than the currently available single-crystal gammacameras (max 500.000 versus max 90.000 counts per sec respectively).

A time-activity curve is generated over an area of interest over the ventricle. A typical left ventricular time–activity curve in characterized by cyclical fluctuations (peaks and valleys) in count rate (Fig. 6). Each peak, or maximal ventricular activity, corresponds to end-diastole (ED) whereas each valley, or minimal activity, reflects end-systole (ES). These time–activity curves have to be corrected for non-cardiac background activity, which can be determined by different empirically found methods.

The left ventricular ejection fraction (LVEF) is calculated by the summation of 4–5 cycles: ED-ES/ED. By choosing a region of interest over the right ventricle, the right ventricle EF can also reliably be determined by this technique. Qualitative information can be obtained by visual assessment of regional wall abnormalities of the right and left ventricle.

Gated bloodpool imaging

With this technique, the cardiac bloodpool is imaged after injection of a radionuclide which remains entirely in the intravascular space. This can be achieved by two methods: Tc-99m tagged to human serum albumin or directly to the erythrocytes of the patient. At present, it is generally agreed that labeling of the erythrocytes provides a more stable tage, which is important when serial studies are desired. Imaging is mostly performed in the 45-degree LAO position for optimal separation of the right and left ventricle. With the use of a gamma camera and a computer system, scintillation data are recorded continuously in synchrony with the R-wave of the electrocardiogram (Fig. 7). Data are recorded throughout the cardiac cycle and stored separately, depending on the relation-

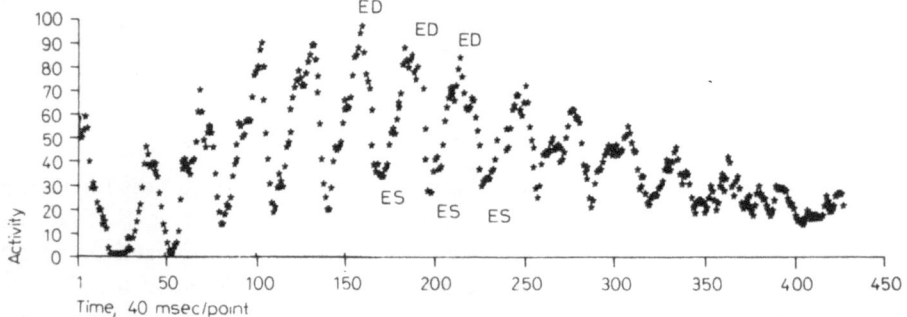

Figure 6. Time–activity curve for measurement of left ventricular ejection fraction by first-pass radionuclide angiography. ED = end-diastole; ES = end-systole.

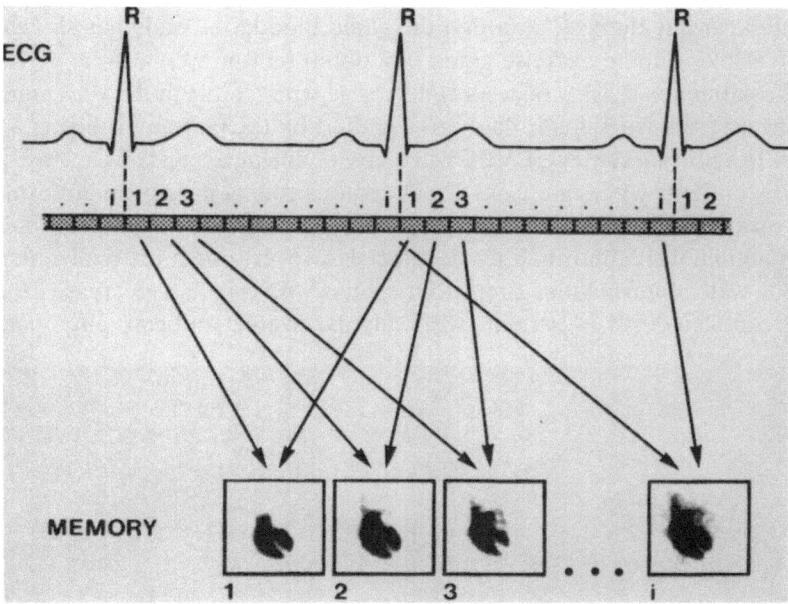

Figure 7. Diagrammatic representation of the acquisition method by which the computer generates multiple gated images. The RR interval is divided into 16–24 frames. The computer places the scintigraphic data of each frame into a memory sequence, depending on the temporal relation of the data to the R-wave maker. For each interval, scintigraphic data from successive beats are accumulated until the average image contains 200 000 counts per frame.

ship to each R-wave. The RR interval is usually divided into 16 to 24 frames. Imaging is continued until 150.000–250.000 counts per frame are accumulated, which takes about 6 min. From these data, a time–activity curve can be generated over a region of interest over the left ventricle (Fig. 8), which shows the activity accumulated over several hundred (300–500) cardiac cycles. The time–activity curve has to be corrected for background activity. The LVEF is then calculated by conventional equation and compares well with the ejection fraction obtained from contrast left ventriculography. Similar to the first-pass technique, visual inspection allows the assessment of regional wall motion abnormalities. However, the spatial resolution of conventional systems is not much less than 1 cm.

When we compare the first-pass technique with the gated bloodpool scintigraphy, both techniques provide accurate data on cardiac function. Which technique to prefer depends on the expertise in the laboratory, the type of camera and specific clinical needs. An advantage of the gated bloodpool technique is the possibility of data collection for several hours (4–6 hr) after tracer injection; serial measurements can be made after physiologic or pharmacologic intervention.

The assessment of LVEF during rest and exercise is probably the most widely used clinical application of the above-described techniques. Both the first-pass technique and the gated bloodpool study are used to evaluate patients with suspected cardiac disease, although the gated bloodpool study has shown to be more feasible. Supine exercise gated bloodpool scintigraphy can be carried out with the patient exercising on a special 'bicycle stress' table under the camera. At each level of the work load, data are acquired by the computer during a 2-min period. In a normal subject, LVEF will increase during exercise by at least 5%. In contrast, patients with significant CAD demonstrate generally an abnormal response on exercise: LVEF fails to increase or falls even to lower values, while very often regional wall abnormalities develop. However, one must realize that only regional wall abnormalities are specific for CAD, since a decrease in global LVEF can also occur in patients with valvular lesions and cardiomyopathies.

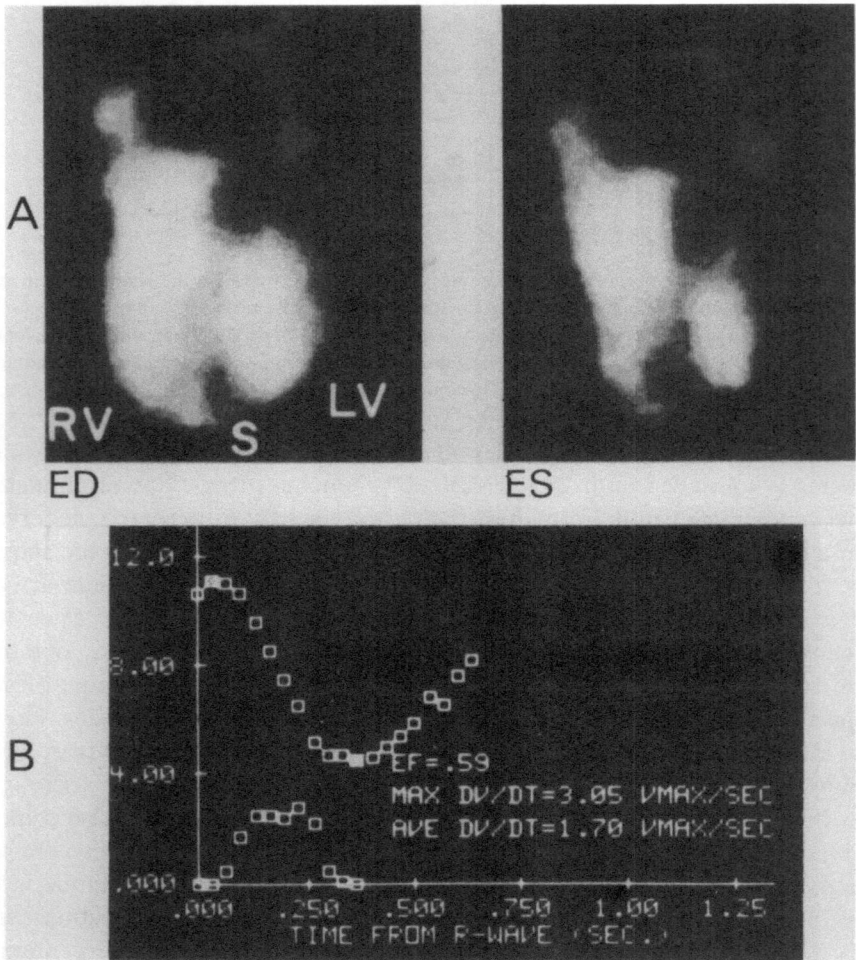

Figure 8. A. Radionuclide angiograms in left anterior oblique view during end-diastole (ED) and end-systole (ES) obtained from a normal subject. The left (LV) and right ventricle (RV) show normal size and there is excellent inward systolic motion of all LV regions. S = septum. B.

Congestive or dilated cardiomyopathy

Clinical findings of both right and left ventricular failure are characteristic of CCM. In general, the pathological findings are non-specific; heart weight is increased, although ventricular dilatation in excess of myocardial hypertrophy is often apparent. Apical thrombi are common in both ventricles and the coronary arteries demonstrate no significant lesions. Microscopic examination usually reveals diffuse interstitial fibrosis as well as foci of replacement fibrosis.

Patients with CCM mostly have biventricular dilatation and dysfunction. Typical examples are alcoholic and postpartem cardiomyopathy, and Chagas' disease. The left ventricle is more severly dilated than the right, and the LVEF is severely reduced (often less than 30%). Right ventricular dysfunction is related to both myocardial involvement and increased pulmonary artery pressure due to left ventricular failure. Wall motion is concentrically reduced, although the apical segment may be akinetic or dyskinetic. The anterobasal segment and the basal septum show diminished wall motion in CCM, whereas these segments frequently show normal wall motion in ischemic heart disease.

Myocardial imaging with thallium usually demonstrates left ventricular dilation and either homogeneous or diffusely inhomogeneous uptake (Fig. 9). Severe left ventricular dysfunction resulting from CAD and multiple myocardial infarctions has been called 'ischemic cardiomyopathy' and may have a picture indistinguishable from CCM. Bulkley et al. [6] have reported the utility of thallium imaging and gated bloodpool scanning to make a distinction between ischemic cardiomyopathy and CCM. All patients with ischemic cardiomyopathy showed a defect on the thallium image involving more than 40% of the circumference of the left ventricular image in any projection. On the other hand, all but one patient with idiopathic CCM showed a defect of less than 20% of the left ventricular circumference in any projection. These findings are supported by the study of Saltissi et al. [7], who clinically demonstrated that a defect size of more

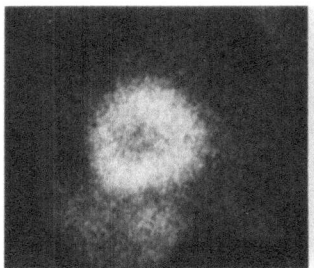 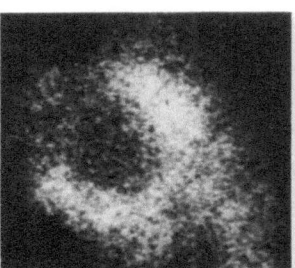 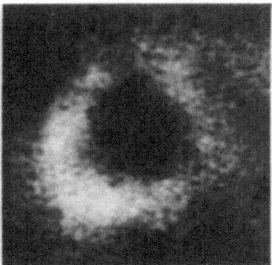

Figure 9. Resting thallium images from a normal subject (left), from a patient with congestive cardiomyopathy (middle), and from a patient with ischemic cardiomyopathy (right).
Note the dilated left ventricle in both patients; the patient with ischemic cardiomyopathy shows a defect size of more than 40% of the left ventricular perimeter.

than 40% of the outer left ventricular perimeter strongly favoured an ischemic rather than a dilated cardiomyopathy.

Also the gated bloodpool scans proved to be useful in distinguishing both entities. Diffuse hypokinesis was associated with both forms of cardiomyopathies, but segmental wall abnormalities were more outspoken in the patients with ischemic cardiomyopathy. Moreover, right ventricular dilatation was more striking in in the patients with idiopathic CCM.

Arreaza et al. [8] showed that radionuclide ventriculography could be useful to evaluate patients with Chagas' disease. Fourty-one patients with chronic Chagas' cardiomyopathy were studied, of whom 12 patients had congestive heart failure. Mean LVEF of these 12 patients was 28% and 9 patients showed diffuse hypokinesia of the left ventricle. From total-group results it was inferred that radionuclide angiography may distinguish the wall motion abnormalities of CAD from those of Chagas' origin.

Serial evaluation of LVEF and wall abnormalities with radionuclide angiography provides an objective method to monitor the effects of drug therapy. For example, in a patient with alcoholic cardiomyopathy one could easily evaluate an improvement in LVEF after withdrawal of alcohol intake and administration of diuretics and digitalis by serial radionuclide studies. On the other hand, it is possible to determine the deleterious effects of the potentially cardiotoxic agent doxorubicin (adriamycin). The treatment of malignant disease with adriamycin may result in congestive heart failure. The gated bloodpool scan showed this toxic cardiomyopathy to be of the congestive or dilated type [9]. Serial assessment of left ventricular performance allowed identification of patients at risk for the development of congestive heart failure and of those who could receive therapy safely at substantially higher doses than those conventionally recommended.

Restrictive cardiomyopathy

Restrictive cardiomyopathy (RCM) is the least common class of cardiomyopathy outside the tropics. RCM simulates the findings of constrictive pericardial disease and shows normal-sized or small ventricles. It may be divided into two basic types of cardiomyopathy; (1) infiltrative RCM, such as amyloid disease, in which the left or both ventricular cavities are normal to decreased in size and the walls are normal to decreased in thickness, and (2) obliterative RCM, such as metastatic carcinoma, in which the involved ventricles are reduced in size and there is partial obliteration of one or both of the ventricular cavities.

Myocardial imaging with thallium may be helpful to depict increased mural thickness, as with amyloid disease, or regional myocardial defects, as with metastatic carcinoma. In case of leukemic infiltration, the myocardial image will display uniform thallium activity since the infiltration is usually homogeneous.

The gated bloodpool scan is useful in distinguishing between CCM and RCM by depicting the sizes of the cardiac chambers [10]. In CCM all four chambers are dilated, whereas in RCM the ventricles are normal to reduced in size but the atria are dilated. In addition, the gated bloodpool scan may differentiate between the infiltrative and the obliterative forms of RCM. In the infiltrative type, both ventricles are mostly normal or reduced in size, wheras in the obliterative type either or both ventricles are generally smaller than normal. However, since RCM is rare disease in Western countries, it is clear that radionuclide data on RCM are very scarce.

Hypertrophic cardiomyopathy

Hypertrophic cardiomyopathy (HCM) is characterized by left ventricular hypertrophy of unknown cause [11]. Hypertrophy is generally asymmetric, with the interventricular septum disproportionally thickened in comparison to the remainder of the left ventricular wall. HCM may be obstructive or non-obstructive. Left ventricular outflow obstruction is caused by hypertrophy of the anterior superior aspect of the interventricular septum and abnormal motion of the anterior leaflet of the mitral valve. Before the non-invasive techniques were developed, the diagnosis of HCM depended largely on accurate interpretation of physical findings.

Non-invasive imaging techniques have permitted the diagnosis of HCM with or without obstruction. Asymmetric hypertrophy (ASH) is easily documented by echocardiography and has been employed as a marker of HCM. However, although a septal-to-posterior wall ratio of 1.3 or more is a sensitive indicator for HCM, it is not pathognomonic. For example, right ventricular hypertrophy may also lead to ASH. Systolic anterior motion (SAM) of the anterior mitral valve leaflet has been shown to correlate with the presence and the severity of the outflow obstruction; this finding may be used to distinguish between patients with and without obstruction. Similar to ASH, SAM is not pathognomonic for HCM and may occur in other forms of heart disease. In recent years, more attention has been focused on diastolic parameters. It has been shown that patients with HCM manifest abnormal diastolic dysfunction in terms of a prolonged relaxation–time index, impaired diastolic filling and increased chamber stiffness.

Both myocardial imaging with thallium-201 and the gated bloodpool scan are helpful alternatives to the echocardiogram in the detection of HCM. Bulkley et al. [12] employed thallium imaging to evaluate the ratio of septal to posterior thickness in patients with HCM. ASH was observed in all 10 patients with HCM and confirmed in nine by cardiac catheterization. In addition, it was noted that the basal and midposterior walls were of equal thickness in patients with obstructive HCM, but that the basal wall was thinner than the midposterior wall in patients with non-obstructive HCM. Three patients with chronic pulmonary hypertension had ASH on the thallium image, but in these patients the right ventricular free wall thickness was equal to the septal thickness, which is consistent with right ventricular hypertrophy.

Rubin et al. evaluated the presence of anginal symptoms in 10 patients with HCM by thallium exercise scintigraphy [13]. All 10 patients had normal coronary angiograms. In nine of the 10 patients thallium imaging revealed no significant perfusion defects and it was concluded that thallium exercise scintigraphy is a valuable method to rule out significant CAD in patients with HCM. The configuration of the interventricular septum on the thallium scan in a patient with HCM is showed in Figure 10.

The end-diastolic image of the gated bloodpool scan in LAO view allows evaluation of the interventricular septal configuration. The appearance of the interventricular septum by gated scan not only depends on septal configuration but is also affected by the angle of view. In a shallow LAO view, the apical septum appears thickest, whereas in high oblique view the upper septum appears thickest. This phenomenon occurs because of the spiral geometry of the septum.

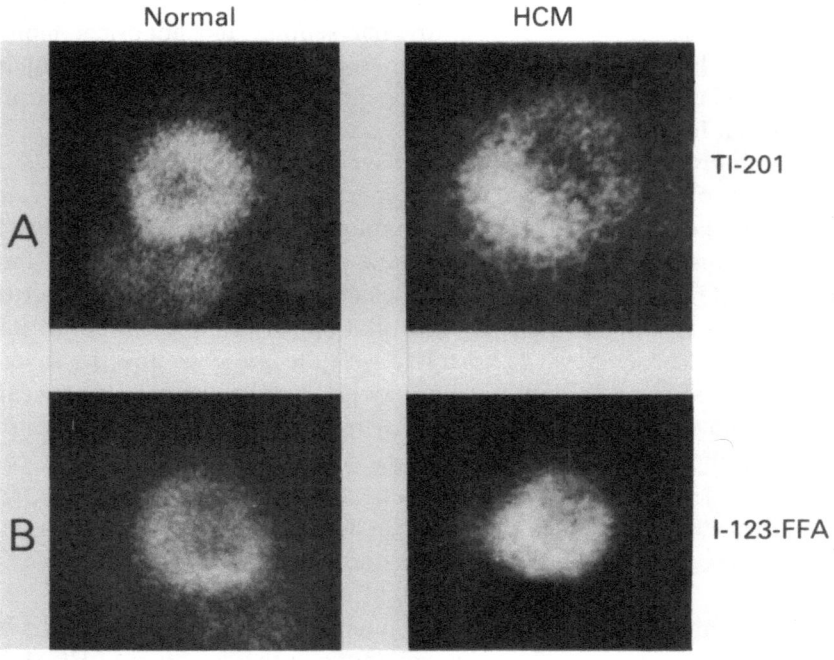

Figure 10. A. Resting thallium images from a normal subject (left), and from a patient with hypertrophic cardiomyopathy (HCM) in LAO view (right). Clearly is shown the thickening of the intraventricular septum. Coronary arteriography revealed no major coronary artery lesions. B. Resting I-123-heptadecanoic acid image in a normal subject (left) and in a patient with HCM (right). Note obliteration of the left ventricular cavity and marked accumulation of radioactivity in the septum.

The most suited view, in which the septum appears most uniform from top to bottom is usually the 45-degree LAO view.

Pohost et al. [14] evaluated 12 patients with HCM by gated bloodpool scan and demonstrated in 11 patients (50%) disproportionate upper septal thickening. The middle or upper septum appeared thicker than the lower septum in any LAO projection. Moreover, 73% of the patients with HCM showed loss of the normal concavity on the left ventricular aspect of the septum. Although this flattening of the septum is a frequent finding in HCM, it is less specific than disporportionate upper septal thickening and can also be noticed in patients with aortic stenosis as well in normal subjects. The gated scan did also demonstate obliteration of the left ventricular cavity and a circular defect in the left ventricular outflow tract. These abnormalities were best seen in the anterior and 45-degree LAO projection (Fig. 11).

Borer et al. studied 63 patients with HCM (40 with and 23 without obstruction) by rest and exercise gated bloodpool studies [15]. All 63 patients showed an elevated LVEF at rest compared to normal subjects. However, it was shown that during exercise LVEF was significantly more depressed in patients without obstruction compared to patients with obstruction. It was postulated that symptomatic patients without obstruction might benefit from inotropic therapy to support systolic function during exercise. In a recent study [16] Manyari et al. studied 19 patients with HCM and 20 control subjects by means of radionuclide angiography at rest and during exercise. The patients were divided into three groups

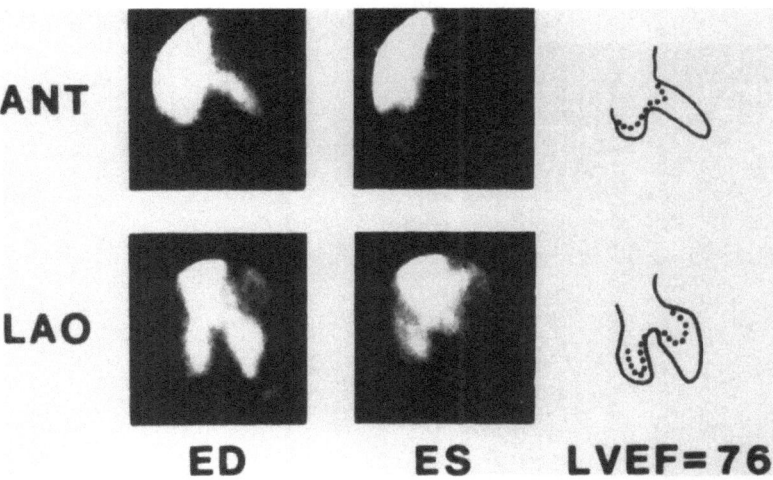

Figure 11. Radionuclide angiograms at rest in a patient with hypertrophic obstructive cardiomyopathy. The septum shows abnormal thickening both during end-diastole (ED) and end-systole (ES). Left ventricular wall motion is hyperdynamic with nearly complete cavity obliteration at systole. Left ventricular ejection fraction (LVEF) is markedly elevated at 0.76. ANT = anterior; LAO = 40-degree left anterior oblique. (Adapted from DS Berman and DT Mason, Clinical Nuclear Cardiology, Grune & Stratton, 1982).

according to their hemodynamic status; those without obstruction (five patients), those with latent obstruction (six patients), and those with obstruction at rest (eight patients). It was shown that the LVEF of the patients without obstruction were similar to those of the control both at rest and during exercise. In contrast, the LVEF of patients with latent and resting obstruction were supernormal at rest (more than 75%). Mean LVEF of patients with latent obstruction increased significantly with exercise, while mean LVEF of the patients with resting obstruction decreased significantly. It was concluded that radionuclide angiography is useful to distinguish between the three hemodynamic subgroups in patients with HCM, and that it may detect impairment of left ventricular systole not apparent at rest.

Bonow et al. studied 40 patients with HCM and used radionuclide angiography for the evaluation of left ventricular systolic function and diastolic filling, and for the effects of oral verapamil (Isoptin 320–480 mg/day) on these parameters [17]. All but one patient had normal or supernormal systolic function, but 28 patients (70%) showed evidence of diastolic dysfunction as indicated by a diminished peak filling rate and a prolonged time to peak filling rate (Fig. 12). Verapamil did not change the systolic function parameters, but improved diastolic function in 18 patients (40%). This study therefore showed that diastolic filling is abnormal in a high number of patients with HCM, and that verapamil normalizes or improves these abnormalities without altering systolic function.

In a recent study [18], Bonow et al. confirmed these findings in 14 patients with HCM and used a nuclear stethoscope for the assessment of left ventricular

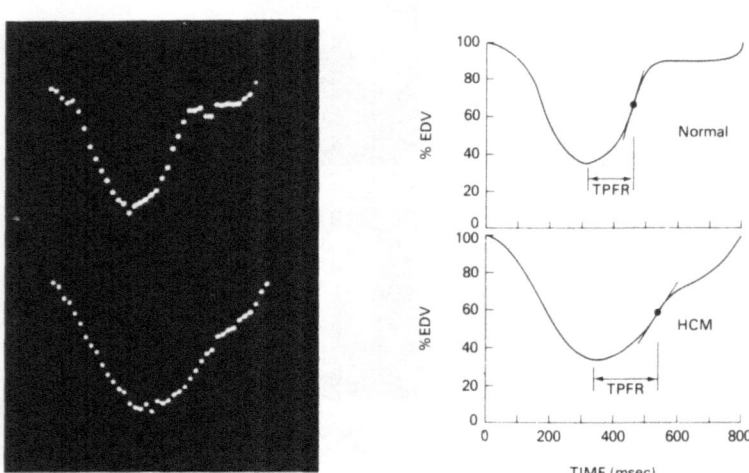

Figure 12. Time–activity curves from a normal volunteer (upper curve) and from a young patient with hypertrophic cardiomyopathy (HCM). The left panel shows the unretouched curves and the right panel depicts the schematic representations of the two curves. The patients with HCM has similar heart rate, ejection fraction and ejection time compared to the normal individual, but peak filling rate is reduced and time to peak filling (TPFR) is prolonged. EDV = end-diastolic volume). (Adapted from Bonow et al. [17].)

systolic and diastolic function after intravenous administration of verapamil (0.17–0.72 mg/kg). It was concluded that the negative inotropic effects of intravenous verapamil are beneficial in HCM patients by decreasing left ventricular contractile function and by increasing left ventricular volume.

Conclusion

Radionuclide techniques provide useful information in determining the diagnosis, prognosis and therapeutic responses in patients with any of the several forms of cardiomyopathy. In patients with pulmonary congestive symptoms, radionuclide angiography may allow the differential diagnosis between those forms of cardiomyopathy in which diastolic dysfunction is the major problem and those forms in which the systolic dysfunction predominates.

Moreover, radionuclide angiography can be employed to rule out potential resectable left ventricular aneurysm, usually due to coronary artery disease in patients with congestive heart failure and suspected cardiomyopathy. The potential value of radionuclide angiography to determine the genesis of congestive symptoms in patients with suspected cardiomyopathy is exemplified by recent studies indicating that a variety of exercise-induced changes in left ventricular function can be found in patients with hypertrophic cardiomyopathy. Such patients commonly manifest pulmonary congestive symptoms, but radionuclide angiography indicates the presence of a normal or supernormal function while the patient is at rest. This finding, together with the appearance of septal hypertrophy and the presence of subnormal left ventricular filling rate, points strongly to a hemodynamic problem based on diastolic dysfunction and indicates the need for compliance-increasing therapy rather than inotropic support (calcium blocking agents versus conventional therapeutic approach, appropriate in patients with pulmonary vascular congestion).

Myocardial imaging with thallium is very helpful to distinguish myocardial dysfunction due to coronary artery disease from that caused by congestive cardiomyopathy. Furthermore, thallium imaging may depict septal abnormalities in hypertrophic cardiomyopathy.

Research with labeled fatty acids in the field of cardiomyopathy is still in its infancy, but preliminary results are encouraging and stimulate further studies of biochemical disorders in cardiomyopathies.

Finally, although these radionuclide techniques can be quite helpful in the evaluation of patients with cardiomyopathy, application of other diagnostic modalities should be considered initially. These include electrocardiography, phonocardiography and other graphic techniques, and echocardiography. In the final analysis, the information provided by the appropriate non-invasive technique might establish the diagnosis and obviate the need of catheterization, angiography and myocardial biopsy. If invasive studies are required to establish the diagnosis of potentially treatable disease, serial imaging studies can be useful to follow the therapeutic effect of appropriate medical therapy.

Acknowledgement

Secretarial help by Mrs A.G. Scholtalbers is gratefully acknowledged.

References

1. Okada RD, Boucher CA, Strauss HW, Pohost GM: Exercise radionuclide imaging approaches to coronary artery disease. Am J Cardiol 46:1188–1204, 1980.
2. Van der Wall EE, Den Hollander W, Heidendal GAK, Westera G, Majid PA, Roos JP: Dynamic myocardial scintigraphy with I-123-labeled free fatty acids in patients with myocardial infarction. Eur J Nucl Med 6:383–389, 1981.
3. Van der Wall EE, Heidendal GAK, Den Hollander W, Westera G, Roos JP: Metabolic myocardial imaging with I-123-labeled heptadecanoic acid in patients with angina pectoris. Eur J Nucl Med 6:391–396, 1981.
4. Hoeck A, Freundlieb C, Vyska K, Loesse B, Erbel R, Feinendegen LE: Myocardial imaging and metabolic studies with [17-I-123] iodoheptadecanoic acid in patients with idiopathic congestive cardiomyopathy. J Nucl Med 24:22–28, 1983.
5. Dudczak R, Homan R, Zanganeh A, Schmoliner R, Angelberger P, Kletter K, Frischauf H: Myocardial metabolic studies in patients with cardiomyopathy (CM). J Nucl Med 24:P20, 1983.
6. Bulkley BH, Hutchins GM, Bailey I, Strauss HW, Pitt B: Thallium 201 imaging and gated cardiac bloodpool scans in patients with ischemic and idiopathic congestive cardiomyopathy. A clinical and pathologic study. Circulation 55:753–760, 1977.
7. Saltissi S, Hockings B, Croft DN, Webb-Peploe MM: Thallium-201 myocardial imaging in patients with dilated and ischaemic cardiomyopathy. Brit Heart J 46:290–295, 1981.
8. Arreaza N, Puigbo JJ, Acquatella H, Casal H, Giordano H, Valecillos R, Mendoza I, Perez JF, Hirschhaut E, Combellas I: Radionuclide evaluation of left-ventricular function in chronic Chagas' cardiomyopathy. J Nucl Med 24:563–567, 1983.
9. Gottdiener JS, Mathisen DJ, Borer JS, Bonow RO Myers CE, Barr LH, Schwartz DE, Bacharach SL, Green MV, Rosenberg SA: Doxorubicin cardiotoxicity: assessment of late left ventricular dysfunction by radionuclide cineangiography. Ann Intern Med 94:430–435, 1981.
10. Pohost GM, Fallon JT, Strauss HW: Radionuclide techniques in cardiomyopathy. In: Strauss HW, Pitt B (eds), Cardiovascular Nuclear Medicine, 1979, pp 326–339.
11. Van der Wall E: Hypertrophic obstructive cardiomyopathy. Evaluation of treatment by invasive and non-invasive methods. Thesis, Groningen, 1972.
12. Bulkley BH, Rouleau J, Strauss HW, Pitt B: Idiopathic hypertrophic subaortic stenosis: detection by thallium 201 myocardial perfusion imaging. N Engl J Med 293:1113–1116, 1975.
13. Rubin KA, Morrison J, Padnick MB, Binder AJ, Chiaramida S, Margouleff D, Padmanabhan VT, Gulotta SJ: Idiopathic hypertrophic subaortic stenosis: evaluation of anginal symptoms with thallium-201 myocardial imaging. Am J Cardiol 44:1040–1045, 1979.
14. Pohost GM, Vignola PA, McKusick KE, Block PC, Myers GS, Walker HJ, Copen DL, Dinsmore RE: Hypertrophic cardiomyopathy. Evaluation by gated cardiac bloodpool scanning. Circulation 55:92–99, 1977.
15. Borer JS, Bacharach SL, Green MV, Kent KM, Maron BJ, Rosing DR, Seides SF, Epstein SE:

Obstructive vs nonobstructive asymmetic septal hypertrophy: differences in left ventricular function with exercise. Am J Cardiol 41:379, 1978.

16. Manyari DE, Paulsen W, Boughner DR, Purves P, Kostuk WJ: Restig and exercise left ventricular function in patients with hypertrophic cardiomyopathy. Am Heart J 105:980–987, 1973.

17. Bonow RO, Rosing DR, Bacharach SL, Green MV, Kent KM, Lipson LC, Maron BJ, Leon MB, Epstein SE: Effects of verapamil on left ventricular systolic function and diastolic filling in patients with hypertrophic cardiomyopathy. Circulation 64:787–796, 1981.

18. Bonow RO, Ostrow HG, Rosing DR, Cannon III RO, Lipson LC, Maron BJ, Kent KM, Bacharach SL, Green MV: Effects of verapamil on left ventricular systolic and diastolic function in patients with hypertrophic cardiomyopathy: pressure-volume analysis with a non-imaging scintillation probe. Circulation 68:1062–1073, 1983.

5. Pressure–volume and stress–strain relationships in hypertrophic cardiomyopathy

P.K. BLANKSMA

Since the disease was described for the first time in 1957, the pathophysiological insights have changed continuously. Initially the outflow tract obstruction was considered to be the most important factor of the disease. Thus it was called idiopathic hypertrophic subaortic stenosis (IHSS). Many other names have been given to it since, reflecting many other aspects of this disorder.

Left ventricular function in HCM

Systolic function

HCH is characterized by an increased left ventricular wall mass in a non-dilated left ventricle. Although the combination of an increased intraventricular pressure and a thickened wall suggests as such, it is not self-evident that this is a true hypertrophy, i.e. a reaction of the myocardium on increased systolic wall stress. Indeed, in HCM wall stress has recently been found to be normal or subnormal [1, 2, 3]. These authors also found contractility to be normal or subnormal. From these findings it appears that the thickened and deformed interventricular septum is a manifestation of a generalized diseased and malfunctioning myocardium. The myocardial thickening and also the dysfunction is unevenly distributed over the ventricular wall, so in HCM there is essentially a regional dysfunction. When the main localization is in the upper part of the septum, as is often the case, the left ventricular cavity is deformed and the outflow tract is narrowed. This anatomical deformation – its site, size and shape – determines the probability of occurrence of an outflow tract gradient during ejection.

Besides this deformity, an abnormal ejection pattern influences the occurrence of an outflow tract obstruction. As shown by Murgo [4], the left ventricle empties more early in systole than normally, so early systolic blood flow is increased. In early systole blood is ejected at a higher rate through a narrowed, deformed outflow tract, so flow velocity may be very high. This causes part of the mitral valve apparatus (chordae and valve) to be 'sucked into' the outflow tract [5]. This phenomenon is called the systolic anterior motion of the anterior mitral valve leaflet (SAM) and causes a true outflow tract obstruction. It also interferes with the normal mitral valve function causing mitral insufficiency, which starts only after the onset of obstruction (see Fig. 1). The murmur starts just before co-aptation of the mitral valve to the septum, and flow decreases while outflow tract resistance is increasing rapidly. Left ventricular pressure shows a second rise, which causes the double peaked aspect of the dP/dt curve. Aortic pressure shows a simultaneous pressure drop, which causes the peak and dome aspect of this

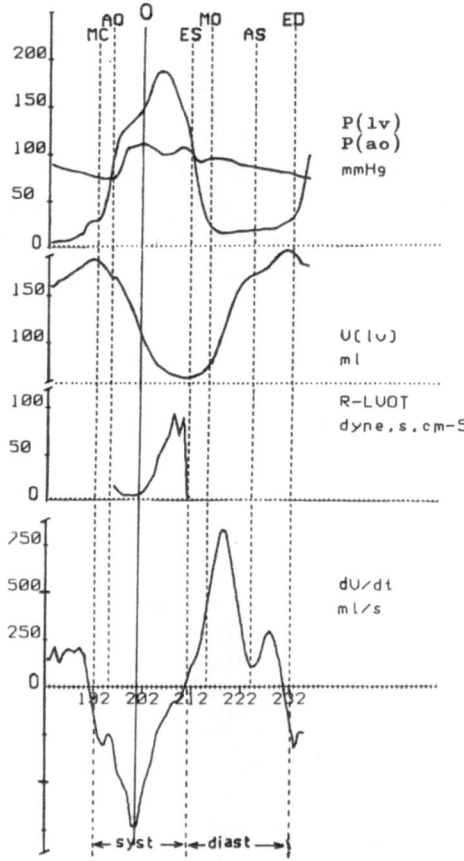

Figure 1. From top to bottom: left ventricular (Plv) and aortic pressure (Pao), left ventricular volume (Vlv), outflowtract resistance (R-LVOT), and left ventricular volume flow (dV/dt). Angiographic frame numbers are given below. At the onset of left ventricular outflow tract obstruction (vertical line 0): left ventricular pressure shows a second rise, aortic pressure falls, outflow tract resistance rises and volume flow shows a sharp decrease. On the left ventricular angiogram it was seen that at this moment the anterior mitral valve leaflet reached the interventricular septum and a few moments later the mitral valve started to leak.

Legends: MC: the first end-diastolic point (dP/dt<400 mmHg/s, the next point having a dP/dt>400 mmHg/s; AO: opening of the aortic valve=maximal dP/dt, ES: end-systolic point=minimal LV volume, MO: mitral opening point=the first point with a pressure below end–diastolic pressure after ES, AS: onset of atrial systole=beginning of increase of end-diastolic volume, ED: the next end-diastolic point (see also page 61 and Fig 4).

curve. The functional fluctuating nature of the outflow tract obstruction is demonstrated in Figure 2. Here pressure tracings are shown of the left ventricle, the aorta and pulmonary capillary wedge of a HCM patient with obstruction that had disappeared after verapamil administration. However, after a ventricular premature beat the so-called Brockenbrough phenomenon is seen: signs of obstruction during one single post-extrasystolic beat with a pressure rise in the ventricular cavity and a pressure drop in the outflow tract and the aorta.

A question which is often raised is whether myocardial ischemia plays a role in this disease. This has been investigated most thoroughly by Strauer [3] who measured not only systolic wall stress, but also myocardial blood flow and coronary vascular reserve (i.e. capacity of the coronary vascular bed to dilate

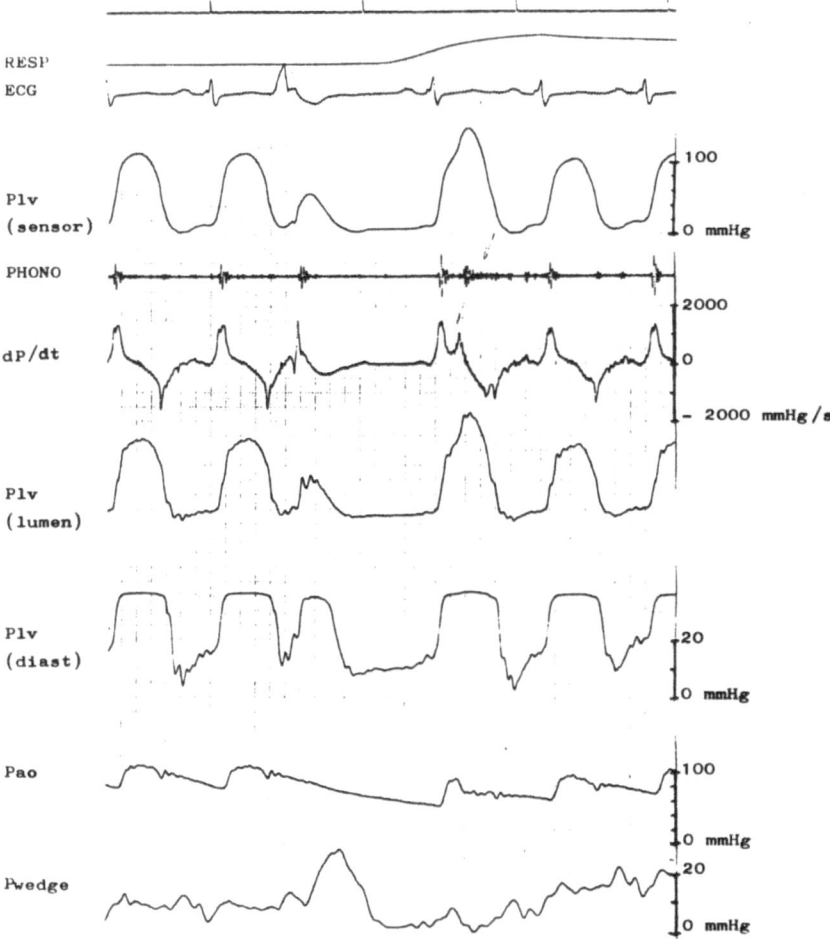

Figure 2. Pressure curves from a HCM patient as indicated in the scales at right. During verapamil administration, the outflow tract gradient disappears. After a ventricular premature beat this reappears for one post-extrasystolic beat, which may be seen from the shape of the pressure curves. During the post-extrasystolic beat also a double-peaked dP/dt (max) curve is present again.

56

further). He found that in HCM wall stress is below normal and coronary vascular reserve is above normal values. So myocardial ischemia in patients with HCM and normal coronary arteries appears extremely unlikely.

Diastolic function

Recently more attention has been given to diastolic dysfunction [6] in HCM. Especially decreased rate and extent of left ventricular relaxation has been focussed. Sometimes this has been attributed to myocardial calcium overload. As there is no evidence that this is actually present, other causes must also be considered.

Recently Brutsaert [7] has discussed the relaxation process extensively in an Editorial of the Circulation named 'Triple control of relaxation'. He mentioned three determinants: inactivation, loading and non-uniformity.

In the first place the possibility of delayed or incomplete inactivation must be considered. This could be brought about by calcium overload. In Figure 3 intracellular calcium metabolism is represented. Calcium inflow takes place in the

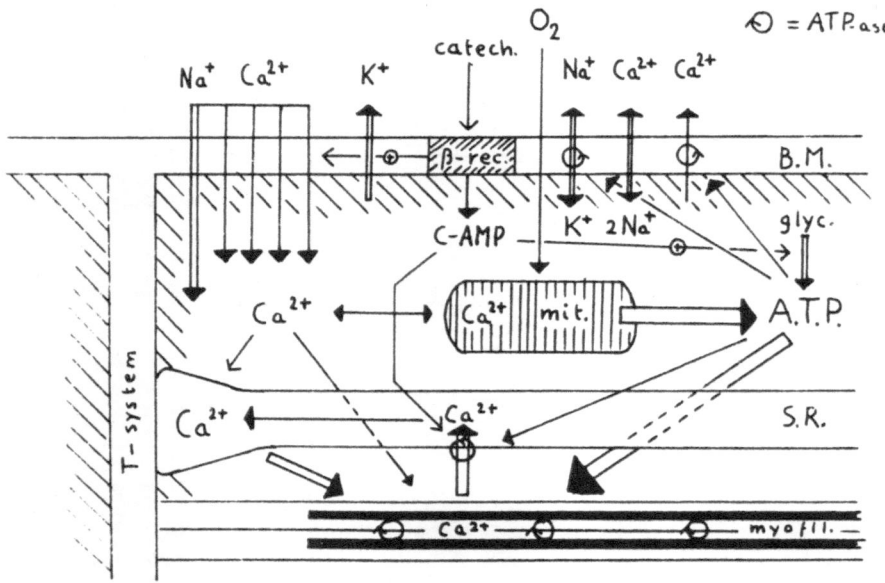

Figure 3. Scheme of the calcium metabolism in the cardiac muscle cell. Calcium enters the cell during the plateau phase of the action potential. It leaves the cell by Na+ – Ca2+ exchange, and the calcium pump. In the cell 4 calcium pools are present: a. the sarcoplasmic pool; b. the mitochondrial pool, in which only a slow exchange of calcium takes place; c. the pool of the sarcoplasmic reticulum (SR), which regulates the beat-to-beat variations of the sarcoplasmic calcium levels: liberation at the action potential and re-uptake at relaxation; d. the pool in the myofibrils, which activates the actin–myosin interaction. The ion pumps, the contraction and the re-uptake of the calcium in the SR are energy (i.e. ATP) consuming mechanisms.

plateau phase of the action potential. The amount of inflowing calcium is related to contractility. As contractility is normal or subnormal in HCM [1, 2, 3], it is improbable that this amount of inflowing calcium is supernormal. Intracellular calcium is further regulated by the sarcoplasmic reticulum (SR) during inactivation. An intrinsic dysfunction of the SR has not been found by Lecarpentier et al. [8]. Ischemia as a cause of dysfunction of the SR or the sarcolemnal ion pumping mechanism is also improbable as we have seen. In conclusion, no indications can be found for the occurrence of calcium overload or decreased inactivation in HCM.

Secondly, abnormal load may be a cause of relaxation abnormalities. High wall stress during the first half of systole and low wall stress during the second half may cause delayed and slow relaxation, according to Brutsaert's theory. As peak wall stress is low, contraction loading is an improbable cause of relaxation abnormalities. Whether low end-systolic wall stress may be a cause has to be established by studying wall stress changes throughout systole.

Finally, non-uniformity has to be considered. This phenomenon is certainly present in HCM as stated before. Most authors consider relaxation disorders in HCM to be caused by incoordinate relaxation [9-11]. In consequence of the uneven distribution of the pathological process in HCM, during contraction a shape change of the left ventricle takes place which reverses during relaxation. By this process the relaxation is prolonged and slowed down. This phenomenon is most apparent in coronary artery disease but could also be responsible for the relaxation disturbance in HCM.

However, the most striking diastolic abnormality in HCM is not the occurring relaxation disorder but the decreased compliance of the left ventricle [12-17]. This appears clinically from the signs of left atrial hyperactivity, which may be found in almost every HCM patient. It appears from ECG, chest X-ray, echocardiogram, apexcardiogram and left ventricular pressure measurement. In studying the resting properties of the myocardium one must take into account several factors.

The function of the heart as a pump may be expressed as the relation of its volume and pressure throughout the cardiac cycle. Systolic performance is determined by the amount of blood which is ejected during systole and the pressure at which it is delivered to the circulation. During diastole the elasticity of the left ventricle as a whole may be expressed as the pressure rise which is necessary to fill the ventricle passively with an additional amount of blood, i.e., the ratio of pressure rise and volume rise when the left ventricle is at rest, i.e., in most instances the end of diastole. But myocardial intrinsic wall properties are not to be derived from pressure–volume relationships, but from stress–strain relationships. Stress is the force per square cm which a part of the myocardium exerts on a neighbouring part. Strain is the myocardial fiber length in relation to its resting length. In the intact heart resting length cannot be measured directly, so it must be estimated by means of certain assumptions. The relation of LV pressure and stress, and of LV volume and strain is determined by the volume/mass ratio of the ventricle. How these calculations are to be made has been described by several authors [18–20]. The relationship between stress and strain is not linear but exponential when at rest. However, when the myocardium is being stretched at a certain speed, stress is higher at the same strain then when it is shortening. This is caused by viscous factors, as is demonstrated by Rankin [21]. He found that viscous factors could have a positive influence on diastolic wall stress under physiological circumstances. This positive influence is proportional to the rate at which the myocardium is lengthening ('strain rate'). Finally, the influence of relaxation on diastolic stress–strain relationship has to be accounted for. As has been demonstrated by Hori et al. [22], relaxation may have a considerable negative influence on diastolic wall stress and could even under certain circumstances cause negative intracavitary pressures.

Drug treatment in HCM

Treatment with drugs of patients with HCM for a long period has been restricted to beta blocking agents, because they were found to cause a decrease of the outflow tract obstruction. More recently, therapy with calcium antagonists has also been proven to ameliorate the clinical condition of the patients. Besides a decrease of the outflow tract obstruction, an improvement of diastolic function – i.e., relaxation – has also been demonstrated by several investigators [23–30]. Incoordinate relaxation decreases according to Hanrath [24]. Early diastolic filling rate increases and time to peak filling rate decreases according to Bonow et al. [31, 32]. They also found, as we did non-invasively [30], a shift in the diastolic filling pattern from atrial systole to early diastolic filling. Diastolic left ventricular pressure and pulmonary artery pressure drop according to Epstein et al. [25]. The diastolic pressure–volume relationship shifts to below and to the right according to Lorell et al. [33]. When given for a longer period of time a decrease of signs of left ventricular hypertrophy have been found by some [27] but not confirmed by others [26].

Pharmacologically verapamil is a calcium entry blocker, i.e. it slows down the systolic calcium inflow through the membrane channels during the action potential. Thus far no intracellular action of verapamil has been demonstrated. It not only acts on the myocardium, but also on smooth muscle cells, e.g., in the peripheral vascular bed. So it has a strong negative inotropic effect on the cardiovascular system; it causes peripheral vasodilation and has a negative chronotropic action [28, 29]. Because the result would be a drop in arterial pressure, a compensatory sympathicomimetic effect is provoked, which compensates for the arterial pressure drop causing the cardiac output to rise and (sometimes) heart rate to increase. Theoretically, verapamil could not influence resting myocardial properties on the short term, because these are not influenced by the calcium metabolism as has been demonstrated by Braunwald et al. [34] and ter Keurs et al. [35]. This has also been confirmed by Hess et al. [36]. Verapamil only could influence the diastolic myocardial stress–strain relationship by improving relaxation and so bringing about a negative influence on stress–strain relationship by means of diastolic suction.

Design of the study

The aim of this study is to investigate *left ventricular function* in terms of changes of volume and pressure, which may be related to the clinical condition of the patient, and *myocardial function* in terms of wall stress and fiber length, which may be related to the intrinsic systolic (active) and diastolic (resting) properties of the myocardium.

Patients

19 patients with clinically and non-invasively proven HCM were investigated by means of a cardiac catheterization to confirm the diagnosis, to establish the functional capacity, and to study the hemodynamic reaction on verapamil. Twelve of these patients appeared to have an intraventricular pressure difference of 30 mmHg or more at rest (obstructive type).

Study protocol

The study protocol included pressure measurement in the pulmonary artery (AP), wedge pressure (APwedge), ascending aorta (Ao) by means of platinum catheters, which maintain their elasticity when they are at body temperature for some time. Left ventricular pressure was measured by a pigtail-shaped angiographic cathetertip-manometer (Millar or Honeywell). This catheter has the advantage of not causing arrhythmias in the frequently very irritable left ventricle of HCM patients. Also by means of the same catheter accurate pressure measurements are possible during angiography. The correctness of the pressure measurement was controlled by comparing the sensor pressure tracing with the pressure tracing made through the lumen of the same catheter. In this way diastolic sensor pressure was also corrected for slight zero deviations, which sometimes occur. For the luminal pressure measurements, Statham P23-ID pressure transducers were employed to which the catheters were connected. After pressure measurements a cardiac output was measured by means of the dye dilution technique [37] in duplo. After these measurements a left ventricular angiogram was made with simultaneous pressure measurement by means of the angiographic pigtail-shaped cathetertip-manometer system. The angiogram was filmed biplane (30 $^{\circ}$ RAO and 60 $^{\circ}$ LAO) by a Philips Polydiagnost-C with a LARC lateral system at a filmspeed of 50 frames/s. Forty ml of contrast was injected at a rate of 10 ml/s in order to avoid extrasystoles and yet get an angiogram of good quality [38]. Film exposure was programmed to lock in on the first frames filmed in order to be able to see on the film the outer border of the heart for wall thickness measurements [40]. Pressure in the LV was measured and digitized simultaneously by a Philips ACS/LVV system. Also, aortic and APwedge pressures were measured simultaneously and digitized later manually. During the angiogram an artificial extrasystole was brought about by a right ventricular pacemaker at 60% of the preceding RR interval. X-ray magnification was determined by filming a 1-cm grid at heart distance. Afterwards, the cineangiogram was digitized by the ACS/LVV system and combined with the LV-pressure measurement. A normal sinus beat was digitized and also the first post-extrasystolic systole and diastole. From the first end-diastolic frame also the outline of the heart was digitized for wall thickness measurements. In this way more data could be obtained of the diastolic pressure–volume and stress–strain relationships. In six patients the post-extrasystolic data were obtained as described above. In nine patients measurements were repeated after intravenous administration of verapamil. This drug was given as a bolus of 0.1 mg/kg body weight, followed by an infusion of 0.07 mg/kg/min. When no clear influence was observed, i.e. a change of heart rate or dP/dt (max) both of more then 10% of control value, the bolus was repeated and the infusion rate doubled. Seldomly another dose had to be given to obtain a definite change of hemodynamic measurements.

Calculations

Volume calculations of the left ventricle were made according to Simpson's rule and according to the area-length method of Dodge and Sandler modified by Kennedy [39] and Rackley [41]. Calculated long axes and short axes from RAO and LAO projections and LV pressure measurements from the ACS-system were fed into another computer system connected to a printer-plotter (Epson HX-20 with a Tandy GCP-plotter), as were the manually digitized aortic pressures. Also, wall thickness as calculated by the ACS-system was fed into this system with the number of the cineangiographic frame from which it had been derived. From these data wall thickness for the rest of the cardiac cycle was calculated, assuming constant wall mass, by an iterative procedure and interpolation. Wall stress was calculated in two ways: according to Mirsky [18] and according to Arts [19]. The latter method has the advantage of being independent on the geometry of the heart. Fiber length was also calculated according to Arts. Volume data was smoothed with a linear 5-point method before calculating its first derivative. Outflow tract resistance was calculated frame by frame during ejection as the ratio of dV/dt and LV-aortic pressure difference. Diastolic stress–strain relation was calculated according to Hess [42] and Rankin [21], using an iterative least squares method for the viscosity constant. All other calculations were made according to standard hemodynamic methods. Finally the computer calculated the following points in time (see Figs 1 and 4): a) the first end-diastolic point (dP/dt <400 mmHg/s, the next point having a dP/dt of >400 mgHg/s) (MC); b) opening of the aortic valve: maximaal dP/dt (AO); c) end-systolic point: minimal LV volume (ES); d) mitral opening point: the first point with a pressure below end-diastolic pressure after ES (MO); e) beginning of atrial systole: the beginning of end-diastolic volume increase (AS); f) the next end-diastolic point (ED). All results were plotted in graphical and numerical way at the printer-plotter.

Statistical methods

Differences were calculated using standard statistical methods: paired t-test for paired data and unpaired two-tailed t-test for other data.

Results

The results of the measurements are given in Table 1. On the left, control values are given of the 19 HCM patients. On the right, the results are given of two groups of patients, who are defined according to the hemodynamic reaction on verapamil administration. The hemodynamic response of these nine patients is represented in Table 2. It may be noted that an increase in maximal early systolic flow is always accompanied by an increase of the regurgitant volume, along with a worsening of the existing mitral insufficiency and vice versa. This increase of regurgitant volume is also related to an increase of the end-diastolic volume, although this is not always the case. In most cases early diastolic filling rate increases after verapamil, measured absolutely, as well as related to the end-diastolic volume (PFR). However, only in group I (see Table 1) are these changes statistically significant. Further, it may be noted that dP/dt (max) always decreases as well as dP/dt (min). Also SVR and outlow tract gradient decrease after verapamil administration. No significant changes were found of CI, Plved, PAP-wedge and HR, although individual variations were present.

In Table 3 the results of wall stress measurements are given. Two types of wall stress curves were found, which are represented in Figure 4 (type A) in which after the beginning of obstruction a second peak may be observed, and type B in which wall stress reaches its maximum before the onset of obstruction and afterwards decreases. The onset of obstruction is defined as the second upstroke of the dP/dt curve. In Table 4 the distribution of these types in the cases with and without obstruction is given. It is of note that in several cases with obstruction,

62

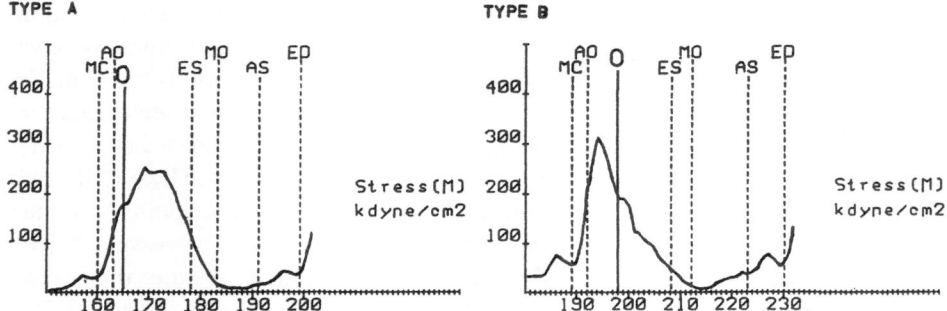

Figure 4. Two different types of wall stress curves are shown: type A in which a second rise of wall stress occurs after the onset of obstruction (line O), and type B in which wall stress shows only decrease after onset of obstruction. Legends as in Figure 1.

Table 1. Pressure–volume data in HCM (mean values and standard deviations)

| | | | Change after verapamil administration | | | | |
	N=19		Group I (N=3)		Group II (N=6)		
Ved	132	± 43	+6	± 29	−25	± 31	ml
Ves	29	± 17	−10	± 31	−6	± 22	ml
EF	0.77	± 0.11	+0.07	± 0.05	−0.06± 0.10		
Vs (b)	103	± 39	+1	± 7 *	−20	± 13	ml **
Vs (n)	76	± 18	−4	± 6	+3	± 10	ml
Vreg	27	± 27	+18	± 1 **	−19	± 6	ml ***
dV/dt (min)	466	± 175	+127	± 26 ***	−135± 83		ml/s *
PER	3.80	± 1.22	+0.66	± 0.17 *	−0.57± 1.32		Ved/s
dP/dt (max)	1386	± 204	−483	± 126 *	−375± 345		mmHg/s *
dP/dt (min)	1150	± 269	−316	± 123 *	−403± 369		mmHg/s *
dV/dt (max)	452	± 185	+391	± 220 *	+90	± 291	ml/s
PFR	3.7	± 1.44	+2.06	± 1.19 *	+1.19± 1.34		Ved/s
Plved	20	± 6	−3	± 7	−3	± 4	mmHg
PAPwedge	13	± 5	+4	± 5	+3	± 7	mmHg
△ P (lv-ao)	68	± 42	−26	± 39	−36	± 27	mmHg *
SVR	98	± 26	−12	± 8	−18	± 17	MNms-5 *
CI	3.3	± 0.06	0	± 0.7	+0.1	± 0.5	l/m/m²
HR	78	± 11	+2	± 19	+3	± 13	/min

* P < 0.05 vs control
** P < 0.005 vs control
*** P < 0.0005 vs control

Ved = end-diastolic volume; Ves = end-systolic volume; EF = ejection fraction; Vs (b) = gross (angiographic) stroke volume; Vs (n) = net (dye dilution) stroke volume; Vreg = regurgitant volume; dV/dt (min) = maximal volume flow during ejection; dP/dt (max) = maximal (isovolumic) rate of pressure rise; dP/dt (min) = maximal (isovolumic) rate of pressure fall; dV/dt (max) = maximal diastolic volume flow; PER = peak ejection rate as a fraction of end-diastolic volume; PFR = peak filling rate as a fraction of end-diastolic volume; Plved = end-diastolic left ventricular pressure; PAPwedge = pulmonary artery wedge pressure; △ P (lv-ao) = peak to peak left ventricular aortic pressure difference; SVR = systemic vascular resistance; CI = cardiac index; HR = heart rate.

Table 2. Hemodynamic changes after verapamil

Patient No.	F (max)	Vreg	Ved	Ped	PFR	dP/dt (min)
1	+	+	+	+	+	−
2	−	−	−	−	+	−
3	−	−	−	−	+	−
4	−	−	−	−	+	−
5	+	+	+	+	+	−
6	−	−	−	−	−	+
7	−	−	+	+	+	−
8	+	+	−	−	+	−
9	−	−	0	0	+	−

F (max) = maximal ejection flow; Vreg = regurgitant volume; Ved = left ventricular end-diastolic volume; Ped = left ventricular end-diastolic pressure; PFR = peak filling rate; dP/dt (min) = maximal rate of (isovolumic) pressure fall.
+ = positive change; − = negative change; 0 = no change.

Table 3. Wall stress data in HCM

Patient No.	Control			Verapamil		
	A	B	C	A	B	C
1	256	260	139	165	−	122
2	138	192	46	137	131	44
3	178	254	118	133	166 °	67
4	330	272	124	328	−	144
5	263	−	206	229	−	79
6	89	235	78	80	176	72
7	128	130 °	90	118	132 °	66
8	351	431	223	156	199 °	93
9	276	292	101	192	224	13
Mean ± SD	212 ± 94	259 ± 81	125 ± 58	184 ± 93*	208 ± 80*	78 ± 35*

Figures are given in $kdyne/cm^2$. Figures marked with ° are measured in the second half of ejection.
A = before onset of obstruction; B = after onset of obstruction; C = end-systolic.
* = P <0.05 vs control.

Table 4. Wall stress curves with and without obstruction

	Type A	Type B
Obstructive	8	4
Non-obstructive	1	6

64

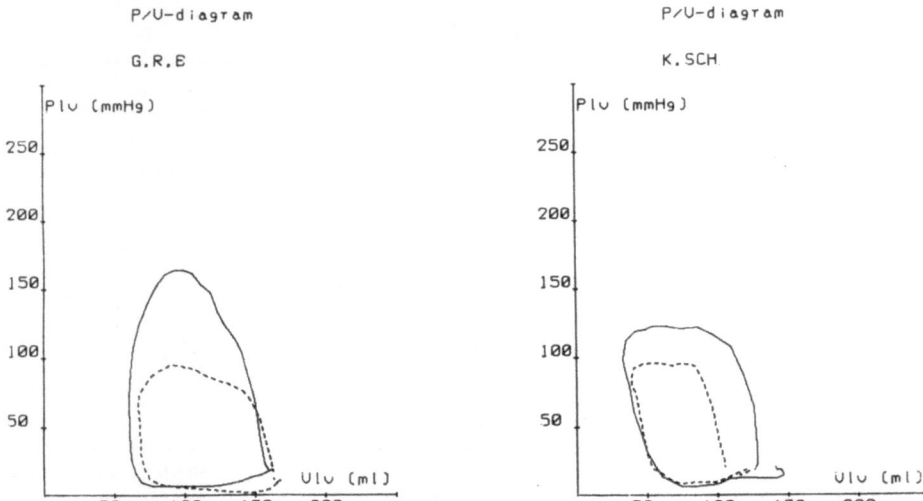

Figure 5. Two types of reaction of the pressure–volume loop of patients with HCM on verapamil administration. Solid line before, broken line after verapamil. At left the diastolic pressure–volume relation after verapamil descends below control level, but finally returns to the same end-diastolic point as before verapamil. At right the diastolic pressure–volume relationship does not change after verapamil administration; only a smaller end-diastolic volume and pressure is reached. However, in both cases stroke work has diminished as is indicated by the lower end-systolic pressure-volume relation and a smaller area enclosed by the broken lines.

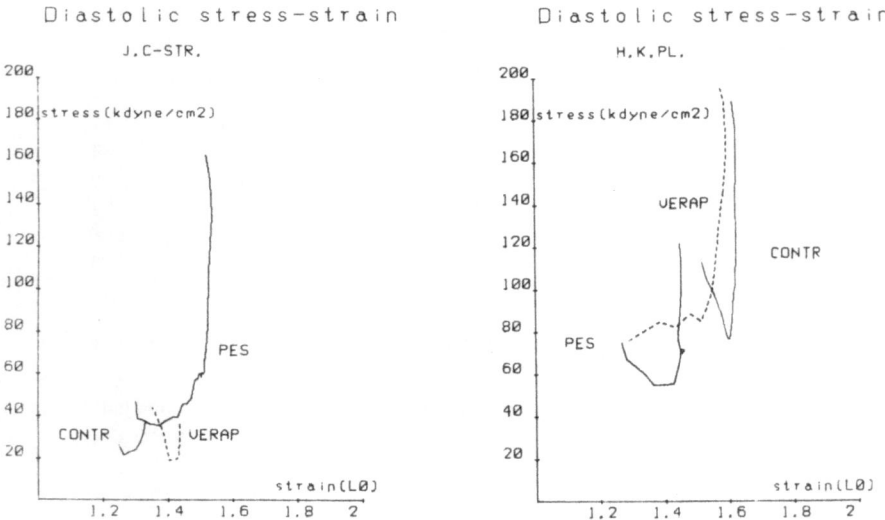

Figure 6. Two types of reaction of the diastolic stress–strain relationship of patients with HCM on verapamil administration. At left the diastolic stress-strain relationship descends after verapamil (broken line) below control values, but returns to the same exponential relationship as during control conditions (CONTR) and the post-extrasystolic beat (PES). At right the diastolic stress–strain relationship after verapamil remains above those during control conditions and the post-extrasystolic beat.

Table 5. Effect of post-extrasystolic potentiation.

	Control (N = 10)	Change after verapamil
Vs (b)	61 ± 21	+ 22 ± 18 ml **
F (max)	327 ± 137	+ 92 ± 121 ml *
dP/dt (max)	1125 ± 270	+ 23 ± 180 mmHg/s

Vs (b) = gross (angiographic) stroke volume; F (max) = maximal ejection flow; dP/dt (max) = maximal rate of pressure rise.
* = P < 0.05 vs control;
** = P < 0.005 vs control.

along with a second rise of left ventricular pressure during ejection, a type B wall stress curve may be found. In Table 3 the values are given of peak wall stress before and after obstruction and at end-systole. All values decrease significantly after verapamil. In some cases a type A curve becomes a type B curve (cases 1 and 4). Those cases in which peak wall stress is measured in the second half of ejection are marked with an o. After verapamil this is found more frequently than before. So after verapamil no definite change of the distribution of wall stress during systole can be found.

For all patients pressure–volume loops were calculated. In two out of nine patients the diastolic pressure–volume relationship was clearly shifted to the right and below after verapamil. In the other seven patients no clear changes could be detected (see Fig. 5).

Also the diastolic stress–strain relationship was calculated. In four patients this was shifted to the right and below after verapamil. However, the end-diastolic point was always on the same exponential line, representing the elastic properties of the myocardium, compared to the situation before verapamil administration (see Fig. 6).

Post-extrasystolic potentiation was applied to give a positive inotropic stimulus and to give an extra volume load. The results are given in Table 5 where measurements of 10 post-extrasystolic beats are given during control conditions and after verapamil. As can be seen, no positive inotropic effect could be demonstrated but an extra volume load was always present. For the rest the results from the post-extrasystolic beats were not different from those from the control beats.

Discussion

As might be expected, the effect of verapamil on systolic function was a negative inotropic effect. Besides that, a distinct vasodilating effect was observed. In most cases the early systolic ejection rate was diminished, which caused a decrease of the regurgitant volume. On the other hand, when early systolic ejection rate increased, also the mitral regurgitation did increase. Mostly, when mitral regurgitation became less, end-diastolic volume also decreased. As the actual resting elastic properties of the myocardium did not change after acute verapamil administration, left ventricular end-diastolic pressure increased and decreased along with the end-diastolic volume.

As described before, early diastolic filling rate increased. However, peak negative dP/dt decreased. In one patient peak negative dP/dt increased and PFR decreased (pat. no 6, Table 2). This phenomenon may be explained as follows: the relaxation abnormality in HCM patients is considered to be caused by incoordinate relaxation, i.e. a non-uniformity of myocardial function, one part of the ventricular wall contracting and relaxing faster (LV free wall) than another part (septum). Verapamil has a negative inotropic action, especially on the active part of the ventricular wall, causing it to contract and relax slower. This makes non-uniformity less prominent, causing a less incoordinate relaxation and a faster early diastolic filling.

Further it has to be considered if an altered load after verapamil administration could cause an improved relaxation. It is probable that a decreased end-systolic wall stress accounts for at least a part of the relaxation disturbance in some HCM patients. However, no evidence has been found that an increase of end-systolic load could explain the improved early diastolic filling rate. Indeed, peak negative dP/dt is nearly always lowered after verapamil administration.

In some patients the increase in early diastolic filling rate was more prominent than in others. The result is an increase of filling in early diastole and a decrease in late diastole during atrial systole. In several cases after verapamil the diastolic stress–strain relation moved towards values below and to the right of control values. At end-diastole, however, it returned to the same exponential (elastic) relationship as during control conditions, indicating that the elastic properties had not changed (see Fig. 6). Until now we were unable to demonstrate viscous (rate dependent) factors in this investigation.

So, in conclusion, acute intravenous verapamil administration in patients with HCM, especially when obstruction is present, could cause some improvement of the hemodynamic condition, although in our patients we could not demonstrate a consistent beneficial effect. No statistically significant decrease of wedge pressure and increase of cardiac output was observed in the patient group as a whole. But in some patients wedge pressure decreased or output increased, while in others it did not or even worsened. This could be explained by a lengthening of the PR-interval or an increase in heart rate, which is sometimes observed during intravenous, but also during oral administration. As pharmacokinetics is probably quite different in these two ways of administration, further investigation is needed to clarify this point.

A decrease in wedge pressure could be caused by a faster early diastolic filling or by a decrease of mitral insufficiency due to a slower early systolic ejection rate, causing a lower end-diastolic volume with the same net stroke volume. Finally the essential changes in hemodynamics could probably also be monitored non-invasively by means of radionuclide methods, i.e. PFR and PER and apexcardiography (contractility, relaxation rate and atrial activity). In this way long-term hemodynamic changes during oral verapamil therapy might also be followed.

References

1. Pouleur H, Rousseau MF, van Eyll Chr, Brasseur LA, Charlier AA: Force-velocity-length relations in hypertrophic cardiomyopathy - evidence of normal or depressed myocardial contractility. Am J Cardiol 52:813–17, 1983.
2. Strauer BE: Left ventricular dynamics, energetics and coronary hemodynamics in hypertrophic heart disease. Eur Heart J 4 (suppl A):137–42, 1983.
3. Strauer BE: Myocardial oxygen consumption in chronic heart disease: role of wall stress, hypertrophy and coronary reserve. Am J Cardiol 44:730–740, 1979.
4. Murgo JP: Dynamics of left ventricular ejection in obstructive and non-obstructive hypertrophic cardiomyopathy. J Clin Invest 66:1369–82, 1980.
5. Henry WL, Clark CE, Griffith JM, Epstein SE: Mechanism of left ventricular outflow tract obstruction in patients with asymmetrical septal hypertrophy (IHSS). Am J Cardiol 35:337–345, 1975.
6. Goodwin JF: An appreciation of hypertrophic cardiomyopathy. Am J Med 68:797–800, 1980.
7. Brutsaert DL, Rademakers FE, Sys SU: Triple control of relaxation: implications in cardiac disease. Circulation 69:190–196, 1984.
8. Lecarpentier Y, Martin JL, Gastineau P, Hatt PY: Load dependence of mammalian heart relaxation during cardiac hypertrophy and heart failure. Am J Physiol 11: H855–861, 1982.
9. Decoodt P, Mathey D, Swan HJC: Assessment of left ventricular filling by echocardiography in normal subjects and in subjects with coronary artery disease and with hypertrophic cardiomyopathy. Acta Cardiol 34:11–33, 1979.
10. Sanderson JA, Gibson DG, Brown DJ, Goodwin JF: Left ventricular filling in hypertrophic cardiomyopathy, an angiographic study. Brit Heart J 39:661–670, 1977.
11. Hanrath P, Mathey DG, Siegert R, Bleifeld W: Left ventricular relaxation and filling pattern in different forms of left ventricular hypertrophy; an echocardiographic study. Z Kardiol 66:483–490, 1977.
12. Van der Wall E: Hypertrophic obstructive cardiomyopathy. Evaluation of treatment by invasive and non-invasive methods. Thesis, Groningen, 1972.
13. Van der Wall E, Bergstra A, Blickman JR, Kruizinga K, Kuiper JRG, Mook GA: Left atrial activity in hypertrophic cardiomyopathy, hemodynamic and angiocardiographic aspects (Abstract 592). 7th Eur Congr Cardiol, Amsterdam, 1976.
14. Van der Wall E, Mook GA: Exercise and atrial pacing in hypertrophic cardiomyopathy before and after administration of propranolol (Abstract). 8th World Congr Cardiol, Tokyo, 1978.
15. Blanksma PK, Mook GA, Van der Wall E: Incoordinate relaxation and end-diastolic stiffness in acute myocardial infarction and in hypertrophic cardiomyopathy. In: MM Jagenau (ed), Non-invasive Methods on Cardiovascular Hemodynamics. Elsevier Publ, 1981, pp 291–297.
16. Spiller P, Brenner C, Karsch KR, Loogen F, Neuhaus KL: Systolische und diastolische Funktion des linken Ventrikels bei hypertrofischer obstruktiver Kardiomyopathie. Z Kardiol 66: 483–490, 1977.
17. Van der Wall E: Hypertrofische obstructieve cardiomyopathie. Hartbulletin, 60–66, 1975.
18. Mirsky I: Left ventricular stresses in the intact human heart. Biophys J 9:189–208, 1969.

19. Arts Th, Veenstra PC, Reneman RS: Epicardial deformation and left ventricular wall mechanics during ejection in the dog. Am J Physiol 11:379–90, 1982.
20. Laird JD: Asymptotic slope of log pressure vs log volume as an approximate index of the diastolic elastic properties of the myocardium in man. Circulation 53:443–49, 1976.
21. Rankin JS, Arentzen CE, McHale PhA, Ling D, Anderson RW: Viscoelastic properties of the diastolic left ventricle in the conscious dog. Circ Res 41:37–45, 1977.
22. Hori M, Yellin EL, Yoran C, Sonnenblick EH, Frater RWM: Dynamic diastolic negative pressures and pressure-volume relation of the intact non-filling canine left ventricle. Circulation 62:205, 1980.
23. Chatterjee K, Raff G, Anderson D, Parmley WW: Hypertrophic cardiomyopathy, therapy with slow channel inhibiting agents. Progr Cardiovasc Dis 25:193–210, 1982.
24. Hanrath P, Mathey DG, Kremer P, Sontag FR, Bleifeld W: Effect of verapamil on left ventricular isovolumic relaxation time and regional left ventricular filling in hypertrophic cardiomyopathy. Am J Cardiol 45:1258–64, 1980.
25. Rosing DR, Kent KM, Borer JS, Seides SF, Maron BJ, Epstein SE: Verapamil therapy: new approach to pharmacological treatment of hypertrophic cardiomyopathy I, II. Circulation 60:1207–1213, 1978.
26. Rosing DR, Condit JR, Maron BJ, Kent KM, Leon MB, Bonow RO, Lipson LC, Epstein SE: Verapamil therapy: a new approach to the pharmacological treatment of hypertrophic cardiomyopathy: III. Effects of long-term administration. Am J Cardiol 48:545–552, 1981.
27. Kaltenbach M, Hopf R, Kober G, Bussmann WP, Keller M, Peterson Y: Treatment of hypertrophic obstructive cardiomyopathy with verapamil. Brit Heart J 42:35–42, 1979.
28. McAllister: Correlation of verapamil plasma levels with electrocardiographic and hemodynamic effects. In: Kaltenbach M, Epstein SE (eds), Hypertrophic Cardiomyopathy. Springer Verlag, 1981, pp 322–331.
29. Singh BN, Roche AHG: Effect of intravenous verapamil on hemodynamics in patients with heart disease. Am Heart J 94:593–99, 1977.
30. Blanksma PK, Pasteuning WH, Van der Wall E: The effect of intravenous verapamil on non-invasively measured systolic and diastolic left ventricular dysfunction in hypertrophic cardiomyopathy. Eur Heart J 2:59, 1981.
31. Bonow RO, Frederick TR, Bacharach SL, Green MV, Goose PW, Maron BJ, Rosing J: Atrial systole and left ventricular filling in hypertrophic cardiomyopathy: effect of verapamil. Am J Cardiol 51:1386–1391, 1983.
32. Bonow RO: Effects of verapamil on left ventricular systolic and diastolic function in patients with hypertrophic cardiomyopathy: pressure volume analysis with a non-imaging scintillation probe. Circulation 68:1062–73, 1983.
33. Lorell BH, Paulus WJ, Grossman W, Wynne J, Cohn PF: Modification of abnormal left ventricular diastolic properties by nifedipine in patients with hypertrophic cardiomyopathy. Circulation 65:499–507, 1982.
34. Braunwald E, Ross Jr J, Sonnenblick EH: Mechanisms of Contraction in the Normal and Failing Heart. Little Brown & Cie, Boston, 1976.
35. Ter Keurs HEDJ, Rijnsburger WH, Van Heuningen R, Nagelsmit MJ: Tension development and sarcomere length in rat cardiac trabeculae. Circ Res 46:703–714, 1980.
36. Hess OM, Grimm J, Krayenbuhl HP: Diastolic function in hypertrophic cardiomyopathy: effects of propranolol and verapamil on diastolic stiffness. Eur Heart J 4: 47–56, 1983.
37. Mook GA, Osypka P, Sturm RE, Wood EH: Fibre optic reflection photometry on blood. Cardiovasc Res 2:199, 1968.
38. Rogers WJ,: Quantitative axial oblique contrast ventriculography; validation of the method by demonstrating visualisation of regional wall motion and mitral valve function with accurate volume determination. Am Heart 103:185–93, 1982.

39. Van der Zwaag H, Van der Meer R, Dekkers AAW: Fotografische aspecten bij cineangiografie van het hart, I and II. Gamma 32: 13–16; 39–44, 1982.
40. Kennedy JW, Treholme SE, Kasser IS: Left ventricular volume and mass from single plane cineangiogram Am Heart J 80:343, 1970.
41. Rackley CE: Quantitative evaluation of left ventricular volume by radiographic techniques. Circulation 54:862, 1976.
42. Hess OM, Schneider J, Koch R, Bamert C, Grimm J, Krayenbuhl HP: Diastolic function and myocardial structure in patients with myocardial hypertrophy, special reference to normalized viscoelastic data. Circulation 63:360–370, 1981.

6. Recent views on left ventricular function in hypertrophic cardiomyopathy: hemodynamic concepts and their clinical implications

E. VAN DER WALL

Abstract. Between 1963 and 1983 personal experience has covered 136 patients with hypertrophic cardiomyopathy (HCM). Age varied from 3 months to 68 years (mean: 35,4 years) with a follow-up of 6 months to 18 years. In 88 patients 114 cardiac catheterizations have been performed. Sex: 62 were male, 26 female.

A recent study of 24 patients has categorically confirmed earlier results of the first decade of study of 52 patients by recognizing the irrelevant significance of the outflow tract obstruction as a hemodynamic burden to the left ventricle, and again emphasized the functional importance of the integrity of left atrial function for maintaining an adequate circulation in HCM. Systolic ejection dynamics were put into the hemodynamic concept of 'cavity angulation', whereas the diastolic filling dynamics were considered to compose the hemodynamic concept of the 'atrioventricle'. These two concepts were used in the second decade of study to readily explain the extreme variability of morphology and function in HCM.

The validity of these concepts was elucidated by pharmacologic interventions with propranolol and verapamil to relieve or eliminate the obstruction, and by the construction of pressure-volume (PV) loops and PV relationships in order to investigate the potential effect of beta blocking and calcium antagonism on these diastolic functions. In 13 patients with obstructive HCM, only the intraventricular pressure gradient decreased, leaving the end-diastolic pressure (EDP), the cardiac index (CI) and the stroke index (SI) unchanged. In five patients with non-obstructive HCM no change in any parameter was observed. Right atrial pacing in three patients also showed only a decrease in the pressure gradient, whereas verapamil in three patients had the same effect as propranolol in only reducing the pressure gradient. None of these agents changed the diastolic PV relationships at rest nor on exercise or during postextrasystolic potentiation.

It is concluded that the presence of an outflow tract obstruction in HCM does not mean a hemodynamic burden to the left ventricle, that the 'severity' of the obstruction is not at all identical to the severity of the disease and that the identity, the severity and progression of HCM reside in the diastolic functional entity of left atrium and left ventricle, i.e., the atrioventricle. For the near future, studies on PV relationschips, stress-strain relations, genetic relationships and left atrial function are needed to further solve the many problems of this puzzling disease.

Introduction

In the period from 1963 to 1983 experience with hypertrophic cardiomyopathy (HCM) in our centre has covered a total number of 136 patients. Age when diagnosis was made varied from 3 months to 68 years. Of the 26 patients who died, 11 died suddenly. In 88 patients a total number of 114 cardiac catherizations has been performed.

In the first decade of study serial cardiac catheterizations were carried out for purposes of diagnosis, response to treatment and indications for surgery. Relief of obstruction to outflow was the primary goal of treatment, with the idea in mind that the obstruction formed a hemodynamic overload to the left ventricle. Beta blocking agents and surgery appeared to arrive at this goal [1], but it soon turned out that both therapeutic interventions did not prevent the most dreadful complication of this disease, namely sudden death [2-7].

In the same period several other investigators reported careful studies in which they could demonstrate that, despite the presence of a systolic intraventricular pressure gradient, systolic ejection was nearly completed in the first half of systole [8, 9, 10].

Doubts arising around the hemodynamic significance of the outflow tract obstruction to the left ventricle seemed to induce a certain competition between minds and centres as to the functional priority of outflow tract obstruction or inflow tract restriction.

Several combined invasive/noninvasive studies in our centre were set up in attempts to unravel this functional priority of either ejection dynamics or filling dynamics in HCM. In the early seventies, at the end of the first decade of study, experience with 52 patients had demonstrated that, for a correct evaluation of the functional myocardial status in HCM, parameters of ejection and of filling had to be recorded simultaneously during cardiac catheterization under different conditions and on provocation. The results of these studies established the conviction that the principal and cardinal feature of HCM is an end-diastolic dysfunction as reflected in a consistent relationship between left ventricular function and left atrial activity irrespective of the presence or absence of obstruction to outflow, and not the extremely variable interrelation between outflow tract obstruction and left ventricular function [11, 12, 13].

Initially having been deeply impressed by the fascinating and intriguing eyecatcher of the outflow tract obstruction, we now became more and more convinced of the fact that by paying so much attention to the obstruction we had made 'the wrong start at the wrong side'. For correct evaluation of the severity of this disease and its prognosis, left atrial activity in combination with left ventricular function had to be focussed [14, 15].

The advent of echocardiography as a routine method in clinical cardiology greatly changed this pattern of thinking by providing detailed descriptions of the asymmetric hypertrophy (ASH) due to disproportionate thickening of the interventricular septum (IVS) with respect to the left ventricular free wall (LVFW) [16], the outflow tract narrowing and the mechanisms of obstruction [17], and the variability of septal morphology [18]. ASH and systolic anterior motion of the anterior mitral valve (SAM) revived the interest for the obstruction to outflow and became echocardiographic determinants in diagnosis of HCM.

The great diagnostic value of echocardiography as a non-invasive method in HCM brought about a diminution in number of the invasive procedure of cardiac catheterization as a diagnostic aid. The accent of hemodynamic studies in HCM shifted from diagnostic to research-directed investigations. Newer techniques with cathetertip manometers, better radiological equipments and automatization of hemodynamic and angiocardiographic data broadened the field of research also in HCM, in which the question as to the functional priority and the hemodynamic significance of the outflow tract obstruction still was present.

Echocardiography recently disclosed the great variability in location of septal thickening. Septal deformity could be present at various levels of the IVS, with important geometrical consequences for the LV cavity.

Combining the impressive results of echocardiography with the data obtained from our ongoing hemodynamic studies, it became evident that a close relationship must exist between *morphology, geometry* and *ventricular function* in HCM. It appeared reasonable to consider this morphologic-hemo-dynamic interrelationship separately for the *ejection dynamics* of systole and the *filling dynamics* of diastole. Two hemodynamic concepts were born: the concept of *cavity angulation* for understanding the ejection dynamics in systole, and the concept of *atrioventricle* for insight in filling dynamics in diastole (see Fig. 1).

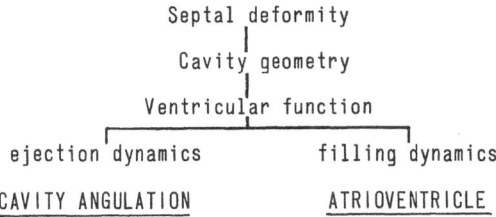

Figure 1. Schematic representation of the interrelationship of morphology and function in hypertrophic cardiomyopathy with the hemodynamic concepts of cavity angulation and atrioventricle.

Hemodynamic concepts

The concept of cavity angulation

The interaction of septal pathology and resultant cavity geometry greatly determines the systolic ejectile function of the left ventricle in HCM. The concept of cavity angulation illustrates this systolic interaction and may give an insight into the variability of the ejection dynamics as a sequence of the variability of septal morphology and cavity geometry (Fig. 2).

Septal pathology dominates the morphologic and functional picture in HCM [19, 20]. The distribution of the abnormal disorganized cells may be more focal or more diffuse, resulting in more focally located septal deformities or a more diffuse septal thickening. This septal cell disorganization is believed to be a post-natal persistence of fetal septal structures [21, 22], and may be considered to

74

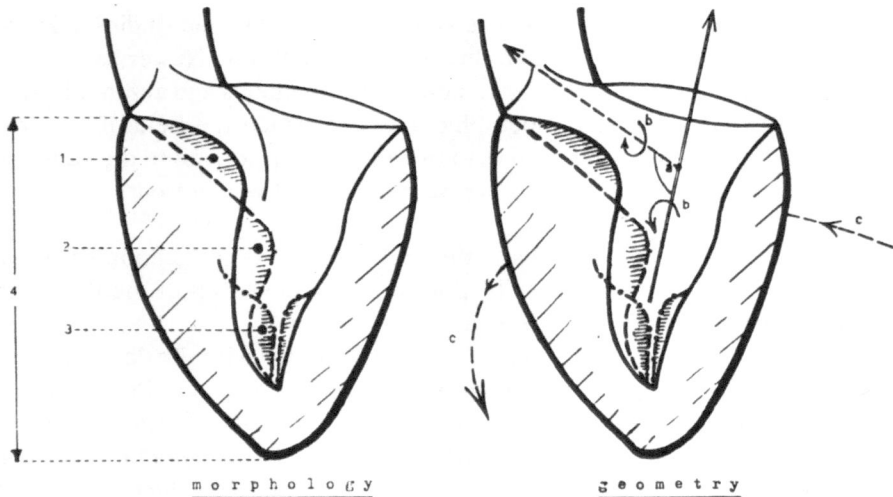

morphology   geometry

Figure 2. The concept of cavity angulation. Depending on the site of the septal deformity the major axis and so the left ventricular cavity will be angulated or not.
Left: Morphology. 1. Basal septal; 2. Mid septal; 3. Apical; 4. Total septal.
Right: Geometry. 1. Angulation of long axis (a); 2. Torsion of upper half with respect to lower half of LV cavity (b); 3. Spatial rotation (c); 4. Preferential flow towards mitral orifice (drawn arrow).

be the primary fault in HCM. Due to the inhomogeneity of septal cell distribution, focal septal deformities may be found at various levels of the interventricular septum. The most occurring sites of focal septal deformity are basal-septal, as described by Teare [23], mid-septal as described by Falicov [24], and apical as first reported on by Yamaguchi [25].

Of prime importance for the geometry and function of the left ventricle appears to be the *site* of the septal deformity. When located above mid-cavity level, as in cases of basal-septal or mid-septal deformities, then the left ventricular cavity becomes angulated, giving rise to the well-known banana-shape of the left ventricle. When, however, the septal thickening is located below mid-cavity level as in cases of apical deformity or total-septal thickening, then hardly any axis-angulation has been observed. So, a focal septal deformity above mid-cavity level opposite the anterior mitral valve may cause a narrowing of the outflow tract region of the left ventricle, the degree and severity of which will be determined greatly by the size and shape of the septal bulge. Narrowing of the outflow tract brings the whole of the mitral apparatus, including the anterior mitral leaflet, closer to the septum and gives this leaflet a position that favors mitral-septal contract and promotes a systolic blood flow now more or less preferentially directed towards the mitral valves instead of the aortic orifice.

Narrowing of the outflow tract also will cause an acceleration of the normal blood flow directed to the aorta. So, obstruction to outflow due to an abnormal systolic anterior motion (SAM) of the anterior mitral valve is prone to occur, either being 'pushed' by the mitral-directed flow, or 'pulled' by the accelerated aorta-directed flow, or both.

The hemodynamic importance of the location and size of the septal deformity may be obvious. It may be argued that the *site, size* and *shape* of a septal deformity determine the presence, absence and severity of the obstruction. In a recent two-dimensional echocardiographic study, Spirito and Maron [26], conclude that 'the size of the outflow tract at the level of the mitral valve appears to be of major pathophysiologic significance in producing obstruction...'.

Briefly stated: the septal deformity determines the obstruction, not the obstruction the septal deformity. Additional abnormalities of septal morphology are a distortion of the septum with an antero-superior displacement of the papillary muscles. Furthermore, thickness and immobility of the septum results in abnormal traction on the mitral valves and a lack of base-to-apex movement. The heterogeneity of myocardial architecture in the interventricular septum and occasionally in the free wall makes the left heart in HCM to a model of regional dysfunction with incoordinate contraction and relaxation. Again, the degree of involvement of the walls of the left ventricle in particular of the free wall, will determine the severity of the regional dysfunction. The major task of filling and emptying is on account of the left ventricular free wall, when relatively spared by the cardiomyophatic process. The disproportionate thickened septum makes little or no contribution to changes in cavity shape and volume during filling and emptying [27, 28].

It is remarkable that the global cavity function appears to be normal or even supernormal, as reflected by the ejection fraction (Table 1). At rest, no difference was found in ejection fraction between the obstructive and non-obstructive types of HCM. In both types of HCM the end-diastolic volume was found to be subnormal. This combination of supernormal ejection fraction with a subnormal end-diastolic volume is typical for HCM and suggests a rapid and complete emptying of a small cavity volume.

Table 1. Ejection fraction at rest in hypertrophic cardiomyopathy, valvular aortic stenosis and normal individuals

	Normal (n=20) Mean ± SD	AS (n=19) Mean ± SD	HCM (n=24) Mean ± SD	HoCM (n=15) Mean ± SD	NoCM (n=9) Mean ± SD
EF (%)	76 ± 6	72 ± 12	80 ± 8	79 ± 9*	81 ± 7*
Ved (ml/m^2)	77 ± 20	88 ± 26	71 ± 23	67 ± 15*	75 ± 20*

Hypertrophic cardiomyopathy (HCM) shows super-normal ejection fraction (EF) with sub-normal end-diastolic volume (Ved).

No difference at rest in EF between 'obstructive' (HoCM) and 'non-obstructive' forms (NoCM).

* not significant.

The conclusion may be drawn that the central hemodynamic fault in HCM is a defective filling, not a defective emptying, present in both the obstructive and non-obstructive forms.

Hence, doubts arose again as to the 'existence' of a true obstruction to outflow and its potential significance for the hemodynamics of the left ventricle. Hemodynamically, the existence of an outflow tract obstruction can usually be recognized by the assessment of an intraventricular pressure gradient developing systolic emptying (Fig. 3). Echocardiographically, obstruction to outflow will be diagnosed when SAM causes mitral-septal contact [19], predisposed by a focal deformity in the basal portion of the septum. The time of occurrence of the obstruction, i.e., the onset of the pressure gradient, appeared to coincide exactly with the onset of SAM, as could be demonstrated by Pollick [29] in a combined hemodynamic-echocardiographic study.

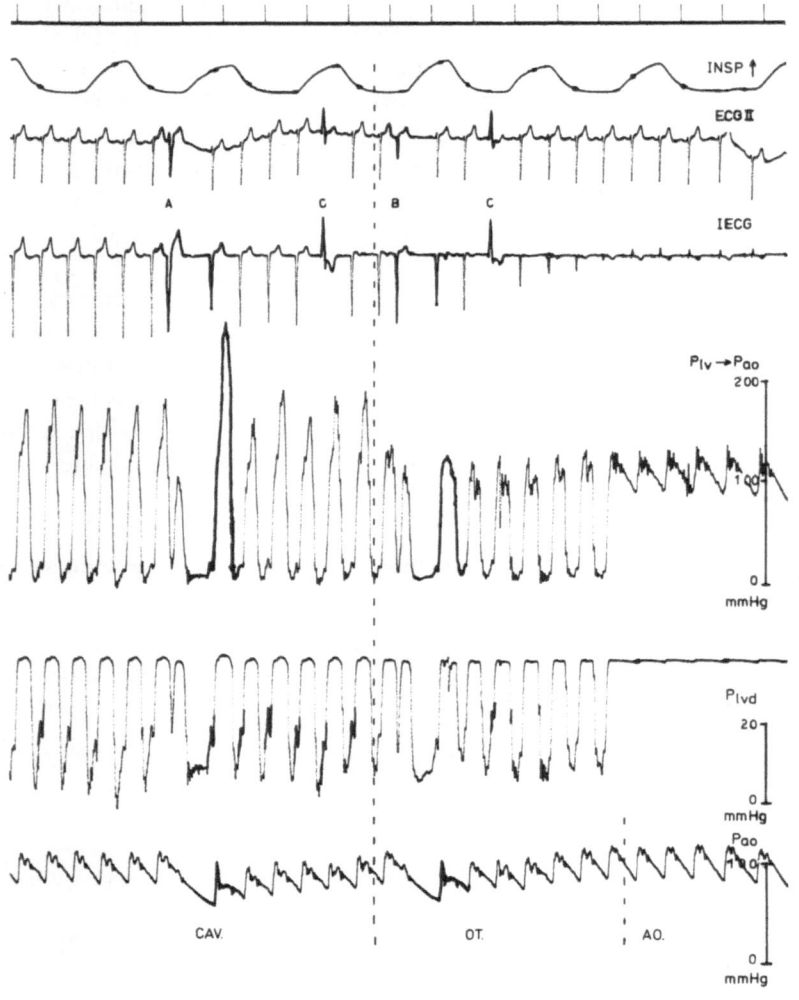

These observations strongly suggest the existence of a true obstruction to outflow. But this is not the point. The point of importance is: if a true obstruction exists, what is then its hemodynamic significance to the function of the left ventricle? Earlier studies of Wilson et al. [30] and recent studies of Murgo [31, 32], have been able to give an answer to this question in showing that the time of occurrence of obstruction is such that about 90% of systolic emptying has already occurred in the first half of systole. Both investigators concluded that – obstruction or no obstruction – systolic emptying is not impeded at any time in systole.

At our institution a recent hemodynamic study has been performed in 24 patients in whom relief of obstruction, i.e., reduction or elimination of an intraventricular pressure gradient, was tried to be obtained by means of the administration of the beta blocking agent propranolol and the calcium antagonist verapamil. If it were of hemodynamic significance to the left ventricle, then relief of obstruction might be expected to be followed by an improvement of one or more of the standard parameters of ventricular function such as cardiac index, stroke index and end-diastolic pressure.

In 18 patients the intraventricular pressure gradient, the end-diastolic pressure, the cardiac index and the stroke index were measured and calculated under conditions of rest and exercise, and in three patients during right atrial pacing in all cases both before and after propranolol. Under the same conditions verapamil was administered in three other patients.

The hemodynamic data obtained is given in Table 2. The effect of propranolol in 13 patients with the obstructive type and in 5 patients with the non-obstructive type of HCM is diagrammatically shown in Figs. 4 and 5. The only change

---

Figure 3. Hemodynamic assessment of an intraventricular pressure gradient in the left ventricle of a patient with hypertrophic cardiomyopathy.

A 15 years old boy with the obstructive type of hypertrophic cardiomyopathy (same patient as in Fig. 19).

An unretouched pullback tracing (Plv – Pao) from the left ventricular cavity (CAV) across the outflow tract (OT) to the ascending aorta (Ao). At rest, an intraventricular pressure gradient of 70 mm of mercury. Relevant beats have been retraced for clarity. Simultaneously are also recorded: time lines in seconds, respiration (insp), the electrocardiogram (ECGII), the intracardiac electrocardiogram (IECG), the high gain left ventricular diastolic pressure (Plvd) and the aortic pressure (Pao). The transition (large vertical broken line) from LV cavity to LV outflow tract is sharply indicated by an immediate T wave inversion in the IECG, as is a common finding. The correctness of pressure measurements is verified also by the normal configuration of the IECG.

The continuous withdrawal tracing shows four ventricular premature beats (VPB). Two VPBs are interpolated (C, twice) and are not followed by a postextrasystolic potentiation neither in LV cavity nor in LV outflow tract. Two other VPBs (A, B) with similar precedent coupling intervals elicit two quite different pressure phenomena. After A, in CAV, the well-known Brockenbrough phenomenon follows with a rise in peak-systolic LV pressure and a fall in aortic pressure. After B, in OT, the same fall in aortic pressure occurs, however – as is usually found – now without a concomitant rise in LV peak pressure. Apparently some mechanism must be present that interferes with the blood flow from LV cavity to LV outflow tract: the 'obstruction'.

observed is a substantial reduction of the intraventricular pressure gradient in the 13 patients with obstruction, whereas in both the obstructive and non-obstructive types the elevated end-diastolic pressure, the cardiac index and the stroke index remain almost unchanged. Likewise, during right atrial pacing (Fig. 6) a decrease of the pressure gradient by propranolol is also the most conspicuous change observed independent of heart rate.

The negative inotropic action of verapamil (Fig. 7) resulted in a reduction of the pressure gradient also without marked changes in the other parameters. The

Table 2. Hemodynamic data of 24 patients with hypertrophic cardiomyopathy at rest, during exercise and right atrial pacing, before and after propranolol and verapamil

		Grad (mm Hg) Mean ± SD		EDP (mm Hg) Mean ± SD		CI (1/min/m²) Mean ± SD		SI (ml/m²) Mean ± SD
Group A (n=13) p <0.01	C	48 ± 24	<0.01	19 ± 5	<0.01	3.1 ± 0.7	ns	48 ± 8
	E	74 ± 25		34 ± 10		4.9 ± 1.0		39 ± 8
p <0.15	CP	32 ± 23	<0.01	16 ± 6	<0.01	2.9 ± 1.0	ns	42 ± 13
	EP	43 ± 17		30 ± 9		4.9 ± 2.5		45 ± 16
Group B (n=5)	C	9 ± 8		15 ± 8		3.7 ± 2.1		52 ± 21
	E	17 ± 9		21 ± 8		6.6 ± 2.3		53 ± 21
	CP	4 ± 6		12 ± 7		3.1 ± 1.9		46 ± 20
	EP	14 ± 8		22 ± 4		5.5 ± 1.9		52 ± 19
Group C (n=3)	C 90	43 ± 11		15 ± 4		3.0 ± 0.5		33 ± 5
	120	40 ± 13		17 ± 4		3.1 ± 0.4		28 ± 4
	P 90	15 ± 15		14 ± 4		2.8 ± 0.4		28 ± 3
	120	13 ± 13		20 ± 4		2.8 ± 0.3		23 ± 3
Group D (n=3)	C	25 ± 19		20 ± 5		3.1 ± 1.6		44 ± 19
	E	26 ± 22		29 ± 6		5.2 ± 1.8		49 ± 19
	CV	7 ± 3		15 ± 3		3.6 ± 1.8		44 ± 19
	EV	7 ± 5		21 ± 3		5.0 ± 1.8		45 ± 20

Grad = outflow tract pressure gradient; EDP = left ventricular end-diastolic pressure; CI = cardiac index; SI = stroke index.
C = control; E = exercise; P = after propranol; CP = at rest after propranolol; EP = exercise after propranolol; CV = at rest after verapamil; EV = exercise after verapamil.

Group A: 13 patients with the obstructive type of HCM; Group B: non-obstructive type of HCM; Group C: right atrial pacing at heart rates of 90 and 120 beats/min, before and after propranolol; Group D: data at rest and during exercise before and after verapamil.

results of this study have shown that negative inotropic and chronotropic acting agents like propranolol and verapamil are able to reduce the outflow tract pressure gradient in the obstructive types of HCM probably by influencing and modifying the force and velocity of contraction and by limiting increases in heartrate. However, this diminution of the intraventricular pressure gradient was not accompanied by a significant improvement of ventricular performance or decrease in end-diastolic pressure, neither at rest nor during exercise or right atrial pacing.

Therefore, it seems justified to conclude from this study that in HCM the presence of a carefully measured systolic intraventricular pressure seems to be of hardly any hemodynamic significance to the function of the left ventricle, not only at rest but also during exercise.

It may also follow from this conclusion that in search of the true identity of

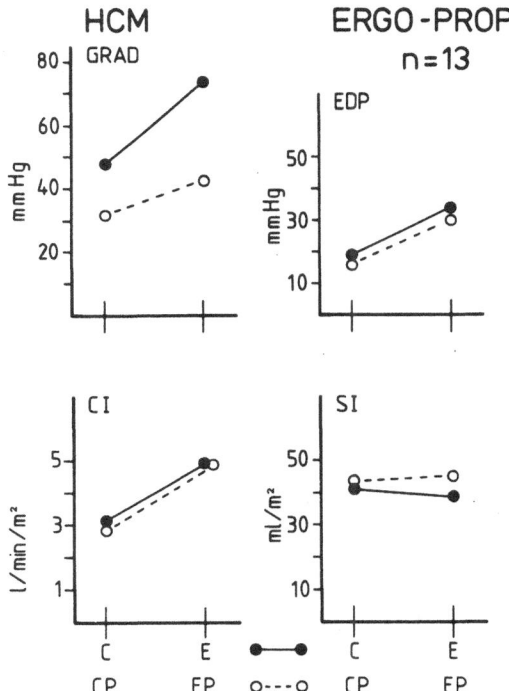

Figure 4. Hemodynamic effects of propranolol on left ventricular outflow tract gradient and standard functional parameters in 13 patients with obstructive hypertrophic cardiomyopathy at rest and during exercise.

Grad = outflow tract pressure gradient; EDP = left ventricular end-diastolic pressure; CI = cardiac index; SI = stroke index.

C = control; E = exercise; CP = at rest after propranolol; EP = exercise after propranolol.

Drawn lines: before propranolol; broken lines: after propranolol.

Propranolol reduces the Grad. both at rest and on exercise. EDP, CI and SI remain almost unchanged. (See Table 2, group A).

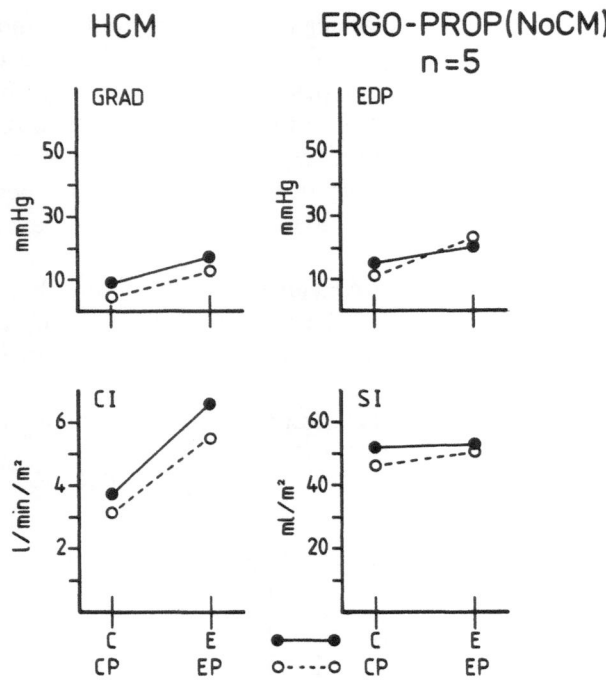

Figure 5. Hemodynamic effects of propranolol in non-obstructive hypertrophic cardiomyopathy. Symbols and legends as in Fig. 4. All four parameters remain unchanged. (see Table 2, group B).

HCM [33] as a morbid and functional entity we have to turn our attention from the downstream phenomena of the outflow tract to the upstream events of the inflow tract.

The concept of atrioventricle

Concept and function. For many years the important role of the left atrium in HCM for the filling of the left ventricle was recognized in our centre. During diastole, left atrium and left ventricle form one open freely communicating compartment with equal distribution of pressure, but with different myocardial structure and wall properties. Within this morphologic and functional unit the left atrium normally functions as a boosterpump for the left ventricle, giving a final stretch to the ventricular myocardium just before the sequent systole by adding about 15 to 20% to the ventricular end-diastolic volume with only a minimal rise in pressure [34, 35]. Asymmetric hypertrophy with disproportionate septal thickening and in servere cases also partial involvement of the left ventricular free wall causes a reduction in left ventricular compliance and cavity size. The left atrium is now confronted with a non-dilated thick-walled left ventricle. It

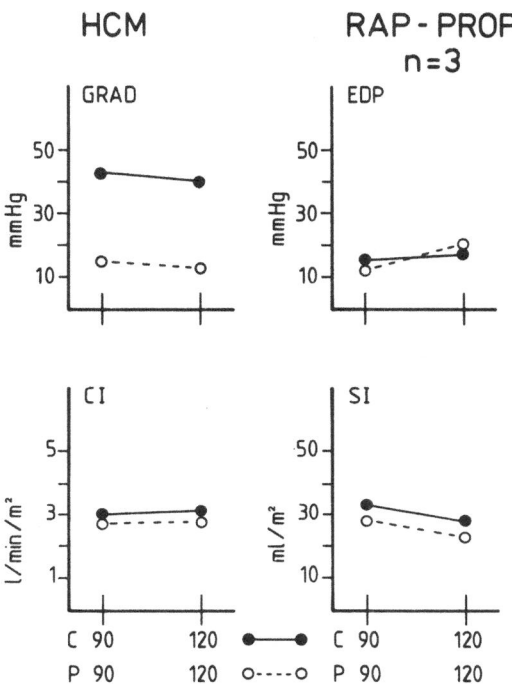

Figure 6. Hemodynamic effects of propranolol in obstructive cardiomyopathy during right atrial pacing. Symbols and legends as in Fig. 4 (group C, Table 2). Propranolol reduces the outflow tract gradient by a direct negative inotropic effect during right atrial pacing at heart rates of 90 and 120 per min. Again, no significant changes in CI, SI and EDP.

is this combination of a non-dilated thick-walled left ventricle with a (non) dilated left atrium and a free atrio ventricular communication upon which *the concept of atrioventricle* is applicable (Fig. 8). This concept is not typical for HCM, but also may be applied to other cardiac disorders with similar hemodynamic abnormalities [36]. Within the atrioventricle, the reduction in filling capacity of the ventricular part may call forth an increase of activity of the atrial part. A gradual rise in atrial pressure now is needed for transport of the blood mass. The boosterpump has become a true pressure pump.

Table 3 indeed shows that in HCM a near-normal atrial contribution in blood *volume,* as compared to that in normal subjects and patients with valvular aortic stenosis, must be expelled into the left ventricle at the expense, however, of an exceedingly high rise in atrial *pressure* of 17 mm of mercury. In valvular aortic stenosis, for instance, with peak systolic ventricular-aortic pressure differences varying from 40 to 120 mm of mercury, the atrial contribution in volume is about the same as in HCM, whereas the atriogenic pressure rise of 7 mm of mercury is significantly less than in HCM. The response of the left atrial myocardium in HCM to this pressure overload initially will be left atrial *hypertrophy* that may

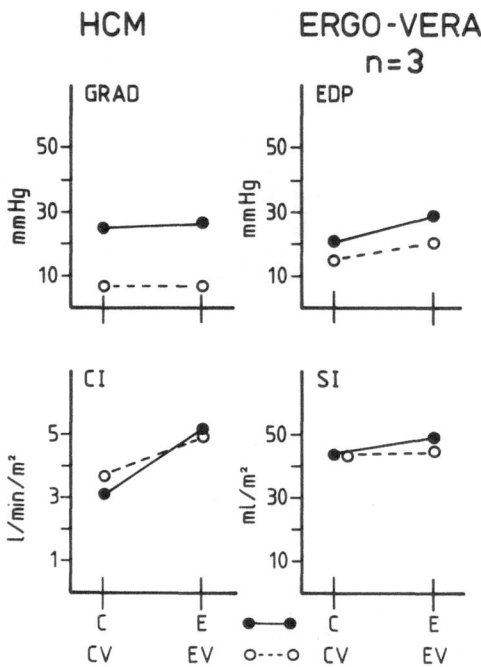

Figure 7. Acute hemodynamic effects of verapamil in three patients with hypertrophic cardiomyopathy. Symbols and legends as in Fig. 4 and Table 2, group D. In these patients verapamil did show the same effects as propranolol in reducing a small outflow tract pressure gradient while leaving the other parameters nearly unchanged.

exist for many years, unless severe or progressive reduction of left ventricular filling capacity with or without defective left atrial transport leads to an accumulation of blood in the atrium with consequent left atrial *dilatation*. Therefore, clinically, the left atrium may be found not to be enlarged for many years, though signs of atrial hypertrophy and hyperactivity may be present, for instance in the electrocardiogram, the phonocardiogram, the apexcardiogram and the left ventricular pressure tracing.

Atrial dependency. Left ventricular filling will become more and more dependent on the atrial contribution both in volume and in pressure, i.e., 'atrial dependent'. Our investigations performed with special attention for hemodynamic signs of left atrial activity have learned that the magnitude of atrial contribution to left ventricular filling both in volume and in pressure is completely independent of the presence or absence of an outflow tract obstruction, i.e., an intraventricular pressure gradient (Fig. 9). This independency of outflow tract obstruction and dependency of atrial function of the left ventricular filling in HCM may further be illustrated by volume and pressure data obtained from three other patients, two

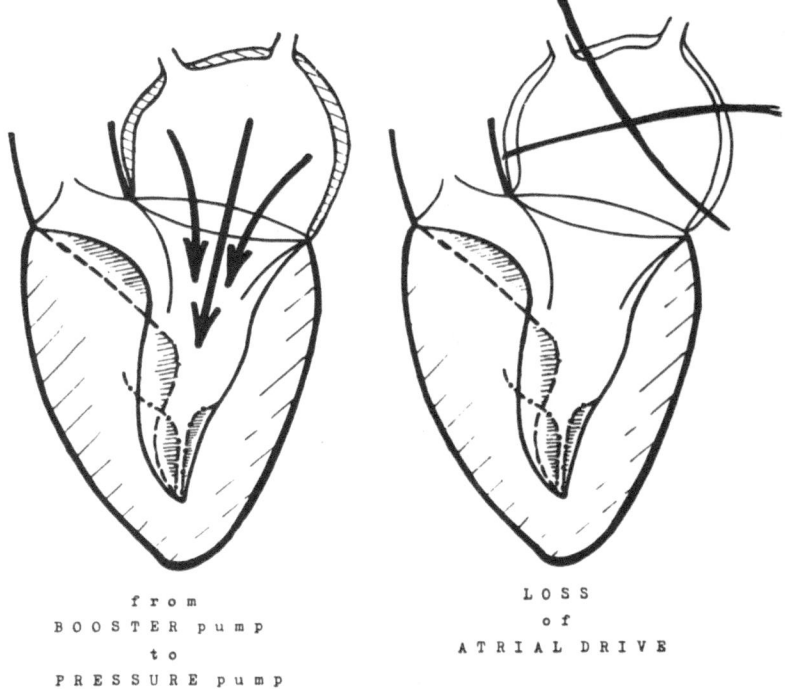

from
BOOSTER pump
to
PRESSURE pump

LOSS
of
ATRIAL DRIVE

Figure 8. The concept of atrioventricle. An inseparable combination of a small thick-walled non-dilated left ventricle with a normal-sized or dilated left atrium.

Table 3. Atrial contribution to left ventricular filling in hypertrophic cardiomyopathy

	Normal (n=20) Mean ± SD	AS (n=19) Mean ± SD	HCM (n=23) Mean ± SD
△ V-as (%)	20 ± 4	20 ± 6	23 ± 9
△ P-as (mmHg)	2 ± 2*	7 ± 4*	17 ± 5*

△ V-as = atrial contribution to left ventricular diastolic *volume* expressed as a percentage of the end-diastolic volume.

△ P-as = atrial contribution to left ventricular end-diastolic *pressure* expressed as the change in pressure from pre-a wave to peak-a wave pressure ('atrial kick').

* p-value: 0.0001.

patients without a provocable obstruction and another patient with a significant outflow pressure gradient at rest. Furthermore, the effect of pharmacological intervention with propranolol and verapamil on the atriogenic pressure rise and atriogenic volume increase will be shown.

84

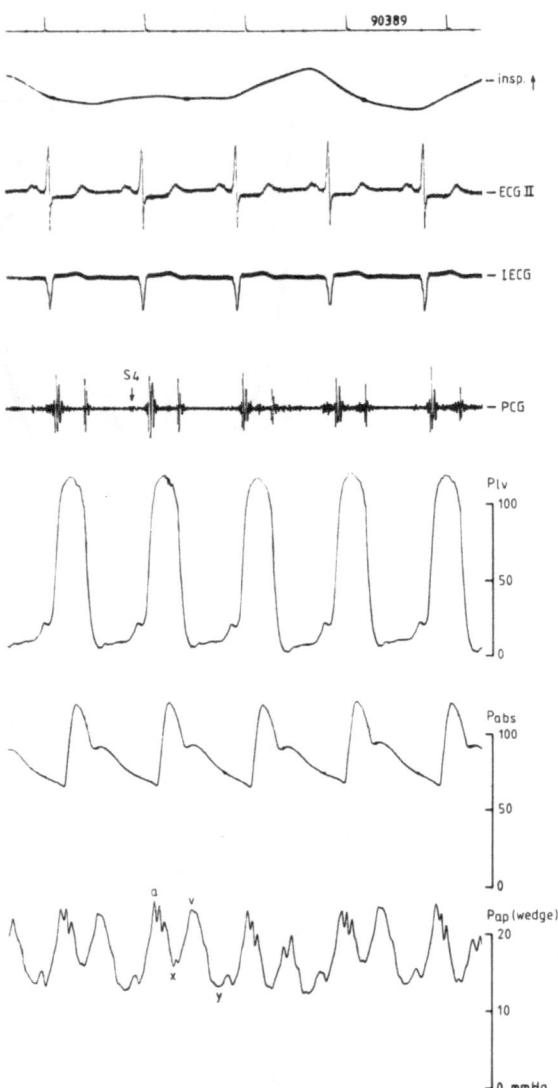

Figure 9. Simultaneous recording of left ventricular pressure (Plv), systemic pressure in brachial artery (Pabs) and wedge pressure (Pap wedge) in a 19 year old man with non-obstructive hypertrophic cardiomyopathy. Independent of the complete absence of an intraventricular pressure gradient both the filling pressure and end-diastolic ventricular pressure are significantly elevated indicating an increased resistance to ventricular inflow. The normal configuration of the intracardiac electrocardiogram (IECG) is a guarantee for having measured a true free-floating endocavitary pressure.
ECG II: electrocardiogram lead II showing a double-peaked P wave configuration; PCG: phonocardiogram showing a fourth heart sound (S4); ejection fraction: 79%. Angiocardiographically no mitral regurgitation

Figure 10 shows a greatly enhanced atrial contribution to end-diastolic ventricular volume of 38% in a young man of 14 years of age without an obstruction to outflow. The angiocardiographic silhouette at b is taken at the onset of the P wave of the electrocardiogram and at c just before onset of the following Q wave. The difference is silhouette contours between b and c, therefore, may represent the relative increase in ventricular volume due to atrial systole.

In Figure 11 the atrial contribution to left ventricular end-diastolic pressure in HCN is presented also in non-obstructive type of HCM. The atriogenic pressure rise is shown in relation to both the pre-a wave and post-a wave pressure and has been measured at rest and during exercise before and after the administration of propranolol.

Several aspects may be of importance. First, the atriogenic pressure rise at rest is already too high compared to corresponding values of normal subjects and patients with valvular aortic stenosis (see Table 3). Secondly, exercise with increase in heart rate and stroke volume greatly increases this atrially-generated rise in pressure to 24 mm of mercury without a concomitant rise of both the pre-a wave pressure and the already elevated post-a wave end-diastolic pressure. This finding means that the exercise-induced additional rise in pressure is solely on account of enhanced atrial contractile force and clearly demonstrates the capability of the left atrium to function as a pressure generator. Thirdly, propranolol is likely to decrease slightly the end-diastolic ventricular pressure at rest, but on exercise this effect appears to be fully cancelled, with the end-diastolic pressure

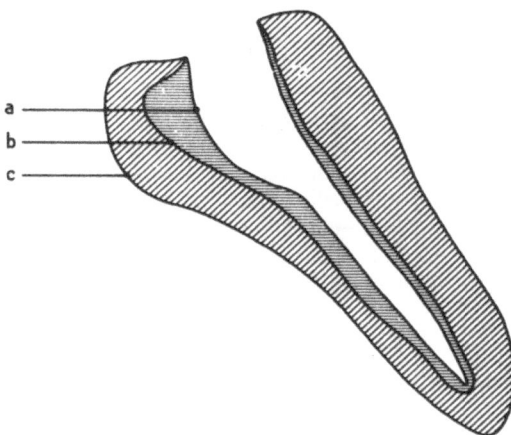

Figure 10. Atrial contribution to left ventricular filling in hypertrophic cardiomyopathy. Male, 14 years of age, with the non-obstructive type of hypertrophic cardiomyopathy. ECG-controlled angiocardiographic silhouettes of the left ventricle (LV), taken at three points in diastole: a=end-systole; b=onset atrial systole; c=end of atrial systole; b-c=atriogenic volume increase.

Despite absence of obstruction 38% of the LV end-diastolic volume is contributed by atrial systole which is excessive.

Of note: the father of this patient was operated for an obstructive type of hypertrophic cardiomyopathy. A twin brother suddenly died two years before.

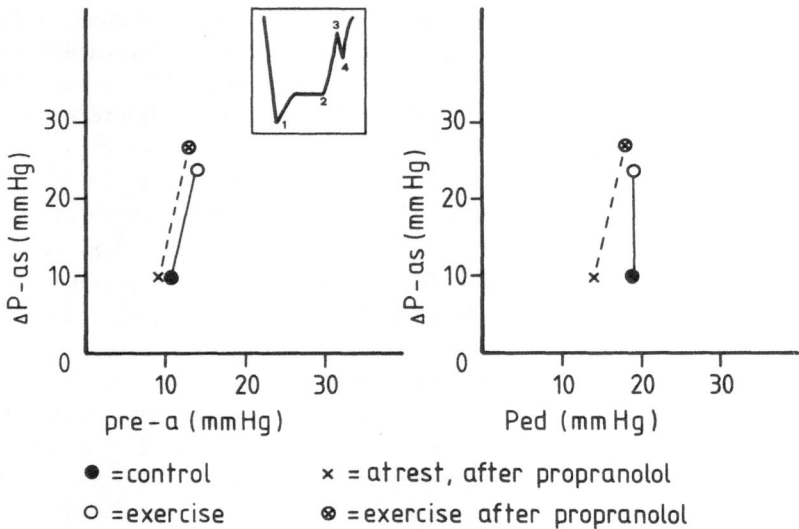

$\bullet$ = control   × = at rest, after propranolol

○ = exercise   ⊗ = exercise after propranolol

Figure 11. Atrial contribution to left ventricular diastolic pressure in hypertrophic cardiomyopathy at rest and during exercise, before and after propranolol. A 19 year old man with the non-obstructive type of hypertrophic cardiomyopathy.

Insert: the four marking points of left ventricular (LV) diastolic pressure tracing: 1. begin-diastolic pressure, 2. pre-a wave pressure, 3. peak-a wave pressure, 4. post-a wave pressure.

Legends: △ P-as = the atrial contribution to LV diastolic pressure due to atrial systole (3–2); pre-a = pressure at pre-a wave point (2); Ped = end-diastolic (post-a wave) LV pressure (4). Drawn lines: before propranolol, broken lines: after propranolol.

Comment: △ P-as is shown in relation to pre-a wave pressure (left) and to end-diastolic pressure (right). The control value of △ P-as of 10 mm of mercury is too high (see Table 3) and is unaffected by propranolol. The elevated Ped of 20 mm of mercury shows only a slight decrease to 14 mm of mercury after propranolol at rest. On exercise a substantial additional increase of △ P-as to 24 mm of mercury is observed merely on account of an enhanced atrial contractile force as the pre-a wave pressure almost remains unchanged. After propranolol the exercise-induced antiogenic pressure rise to 27 mm of mercury is even greater than before propranolol and shows a return of the Ped to its previous elevated pressure of 20 mm of mercury. End-diastolic left ventricular pressure has in large measure become 'atrial dependent' due to reduced left ventricular compliance which is not affected by propranolol.

returning to its previously elevated level of 20 mm of mercury. So, in this patient, propranolol did not affect the magnitude of the atriogenic pressure rise, apparently because propranolol does not improve the ventricular diastolic compliance. When the first derivative of the atriogenic pressure rise of the ventricular diastolic pressure is analyzed (Fig. 12), then the effect of propranolol on the mechanical activity of the left atrium becomes manifest and turns out to consist of a reduction in the *rate* of the atriogenic pressure development, a direct negative inotropic effect of propranolol on the left atrial myocardium.

These observations clearly demonstrate that an extremely hyperactive left atrium may be present in the absence of any systolic intraventricular pressure

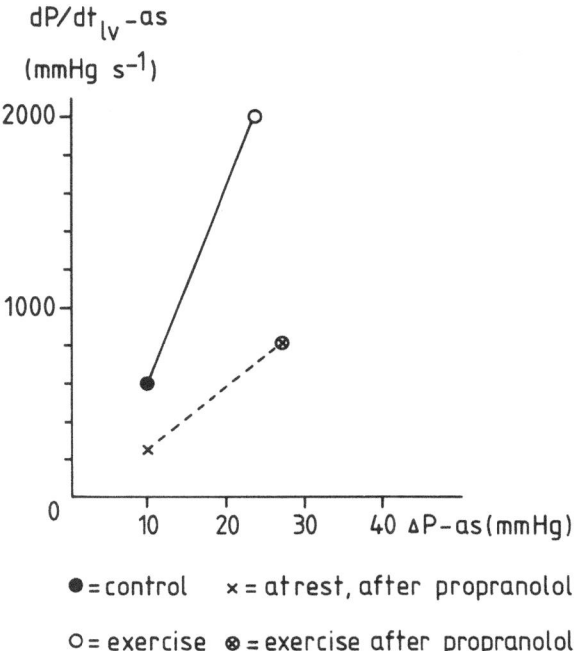

●= control   × = at rest, after propranolol

○= exercise ⊗ = exercise after propranolol

Figure 12. Effect of propranolol on the rate of atriogenic ventricular pressure rise.

Same patient as in Fig. 11. The first derivative of the atriogenic pressure rise of the left ventricular diastolic pressure tracing (dP/dt-lv-as) is shown in relation to the magnitude of the atriogenic pressure rise ($\triangle$ P-as). Each point is a mean of 10 measurements taken in the end-expiratory phase.

After propranolol (broken line) $\triangle$ P-as remains unchanged and elevated, as already has been shown in Fig. 11, however, with a decrease in the rate of atriogenic pressure development of 600 to about 200 mm of mercury per second. The exercise-induced excessive increase in rate of pressure development to 2000 mm of mercury per second before propranolol is significantly lowered by propranolol to 800 mm of mercury per second.

So, by its negative inoptropic effect on the left atrial myocardium, propranolol substantially reduces the *rate* of the atriogenic pressure rise, not its magnitude.

gradient. These observations may allow the conclusion that the resistance to ventricular inflow is responsible for this atrial hyperfunction, not a resistance to ventricular outflow.

In Figure 13 the pressure-volume (PV) loops and diastolic PV relationship are shown of 38 year old woman with a significant outflow tract pressure gradient at rest. In the diastolic PV relationship there is difference between the first sinus beat and the nodal beat of 16 mm of mercury of the end-diastolic pressure (Ped) and 16 ml of volume of the end-diastolic volume (Ved). This finding clearly illustrates the atrial contribution to both the ventricular end-diastolic pressure and the end-diastolic volume. The very small decrease in end-diastolic volume associated with a very large decrease in pressure indicates that the left ventricular compliance in this patient has been considerably reduced. The effects of verapa-

88

mil are two-fold: a marked reduction of the peak systolic pressure as presented in the PV loop (broken line), and also a marked decrease in end-diastolic pressure as shown in the diastolic PV relation. However, this decrease in end-diastolic pressure is not accompanied by an increase but by a decrease in end-diastolic volume in such a way that the PV relation has closely followed the passive diastolic pressure-volume curve. No shift rightward and downward is seen as possible evidence of an improvement in left ventricular compliance. Blanksma in our laboratory [37] and other investigators such as Bonow [38, 39], Ten Cate [40] and Hanrath [41] in studying pressure-volume relations in HCM also have been unable to assess a well-defined acute effect of verapamil on the diastolic PV relations.

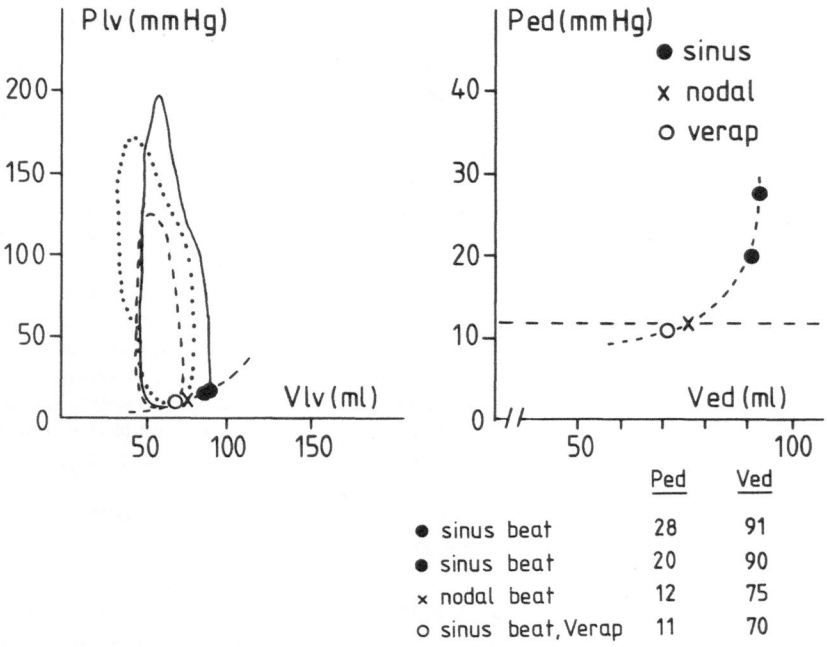

		Ped	Ved
●	sinus beat	28	91
●	sinus beat	20	90
×	nodal beat	12	75
○	sinus beat, Verap	11	70

Figure 13. Atrial contribution to left ventricular filling in both volume and pressure.
A 38 year old woman with obstructive hypertrophic cardiomyopathy.
Left: Pressure-volume loops during a sinus beat (●), a nodal beat (X) and after verapamil (○).
Right: Diastolic pressure-volume relationship taken from this PV loops and magnified.
When atrial contribution to left ventricular filling is abruptly halted, as in case of the spontaneously occurring nodal beat, then both the end-diastolic pressure and end-diastolic volume show a decrease of 16 mm of mercury and of 16 ml in volume respectively, from the first sinus beat to the nodal beat.
The diastolic PV relation closely follows the steep part of the passive diastolic PV-curve. This greatly reduced ventricular compliance requires a greatly increased atrial contribution in both volume and pressure.
Note: after verapamil no rightward and downward shift of the diastolic compliance curve is seen.

Atrial pump failure. When the integrity of left atrial function is disturbed by electrical and/or mechanical defects, i.e., rhythm disturbances or depressed contractile function, then this 'loss of atrial drive' can result in the clinical picture of what might be called 'atrial pump failure' (Fig. 14). Clinically, almost any heart disease may end in a systolic ventricular pump failure with pulmonary capillary hypertension and systemic venous congestion. Visceral and peripheral edema then complete the clinical picture of a congestive heart failure.

In contrast, in HCM the full-blown clinical picture of congestive heart failure rarely if ever is seen. The clinical picture in HCM that usually is called 'congestive heart failure' is, however, dominated by easily occurring and frequently progressive dyspnoea long before systemic congestion could have occurred. As has been shown in the preceding chapter, the left atrium in HCM is forced to act primarily as a pressure pump, which in this context means that a defective pressure transmission from left atrium to left ventricle will rapidly result in a steep rise in pressure backwards into the pulmonary circulation. Rapidity and magnitude of development of this backpressure effect are believed to determine the severity and progression of dyspnoea with pulmonary edema, frequently with a fatal outcome. Therefore, especially in HCM, any clinical deterioration due to defective atrial pump function must be treated as an emergency. An attack of atrial fibrillation, for instance, may be a life-threatening situation, as is common clini-

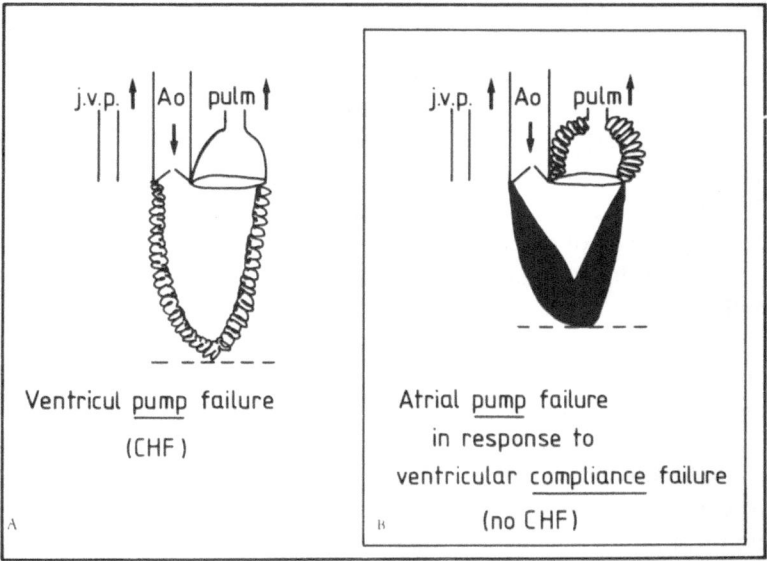

Figure 14. Atrial pump failure. Atrial pump failure: a term to indicate that the clinical condition with signs and symptoms of pulmonary hypertension and congestion is mainly due to failure of atrial transport function in stead of ventricular pump function. In both conditions pulmonary vascular and jugular venous pressures (j.v.p.) may be elevated, however, in atrial pump failure rarely if ever with signs of visceral congestion and peripheral edema, i.e. with overt congestive heart failure (CHF).

cal experience. I believe this to be just typical for HCM, for there is hardly any other heart disease in which a bout of atrial fibrillation can so rapidly result in such a severe and life-threatening clinical situation. Two examples of atrial pump failure may be given.

Figure 15 shows an example of atrial pump failure in a 44 year old man, known for years to have a non-obstructive type of HCM. Cessation of atrial transport has been caused by an atrioventricular nodal rhythm resulting in extreme dyspnoea with pulmonary edema. The backpressure effect associated with exceedingly high pressures in the pulmonary artery and right atrium might be however in this case of a functional rhythm not exclusively due to the loss of mechanical atrial drive but also to an improper temporal sequence of atrio ventricular excitation, i.e. in terms of pressure a sustained canon-wave effect. Nevertheless, this dual cause of pulmonary hypertension turned out to be lethal to this patient during a sequent attack of AV nodal rhythm. Although no full-proof hemodynamic evidence of defective atrial pump function as the only lethal cause may be given, it is likely that the fatal rise in pulmonary pressure has been mainly due to the loss of atrial drive, i.e. atrial pump failure. There is no other reason for this patient to acutely die during an episode of AV nodal rhythm.

Figure 16 shows a less severe situation of transient atrial pump failure occurring during a cardiac catheterization after the administration of propranolol. After propranolol a loss of mechanical atrial activity was noted with complete disappearance of both the atrial kick from the left ventricular pressure tracing and the fourth heart sound from the phonocardiogram. The patient became acutely dyspneic and hypotensive. Propranolol was supposed to have completely depressed left atrial myocardial contractile function by its negative inotropic action (see also Fig. 12). The heart rate went up, whereas stroke volume decreased remarkably with the normal percentage of atrial contribution to the end-diastolic volume, i.e., 18%, as a manifestation of loss of atrial transport function. An interesting aspect of this case report is the fact that loss of mechanical atrial activity occurred during a strictly regular rhythm and not during an atrial tachyarrhythmia such as atrial fibrillation.

Atrio protection. In patients with HCM the integrity of left atrial function, operating as a component of the atrioventricle and an intermediate between pulmonary circulation and left ventricle, may be of vital importance. Preservation of this functional integrity by any method of treatment might be called 'atrioprotection'. On the one hand, maintaining or restoring normal sinus rhythm may be a form of atrioprotection; on the other hand, improvement of diastolic filling by improving the reduced compliance, or enlargement of the ventricular cavity may be considered as factors that are capable of unloading an overloaded left atrium.

The results of our hemodynamic studies have repeatedly confirmed our earlier conception that the cardinal hemodynamic feature of HCM is resistant to ventricular inflow. However, the existence and severity of this ventricular inflow impediment must always be evaluated in conjunction with the corresponding reactions of the left atrium.

Therefore, in our belief, the identity of HCM as a morbid entity may be described as an atrioventricle with incidental cavity angulation.

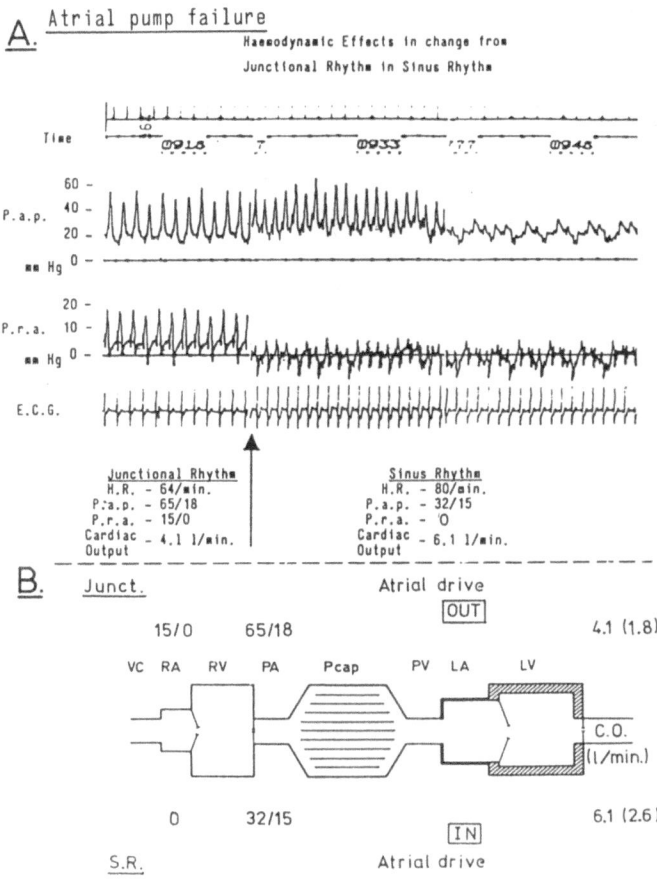

Figure 15. Atrial pump failure in hypertrophic cardiomyopathy due to a junctional rhythm.

A 44 year old man was hospitalized presenting with severe progressive dyspnoea and a junctional rhythm (panel A). Spontaneous transition in to sinusrhythm (at arrow) resulted in a marked clinical improvement. Hemodynamically a rapid fall to normal of the excessive elevated pressures in the pulmonary artery (P.a.p.) and the right atrium (P.r.a.) was accompanied by a nearly fifty percent increase in cardiac output. Stroke volume increased with 18% which is normal.

Panel B: schematic illustration of the hemodynamic changes in the compartments involved when atrial drive is 'out' and 'in'. The tremendous rise in pulmonary artery and even right atrial pressure when atrial drive is 'out' represents a back-pressure effect and is unlikely to be ascribed solely to the improperly timed atrial activation. A few hours after this recording had been made this patient died suddenly in an attack of extreme dyspnoea with pulmonary edema.

Clinical implications

The appreciation of the role of the obstruction in diagnosis and treatment will be a reflection of the concepts described. In clinical practice the diagnosis of an obstruction to outflow in HCM is commonly recognized by the presence of a SAM combined with ASH echocardiographically or an intraventricular pressure gradient hemodynamically. We have tried to demonstrate that the presence of an

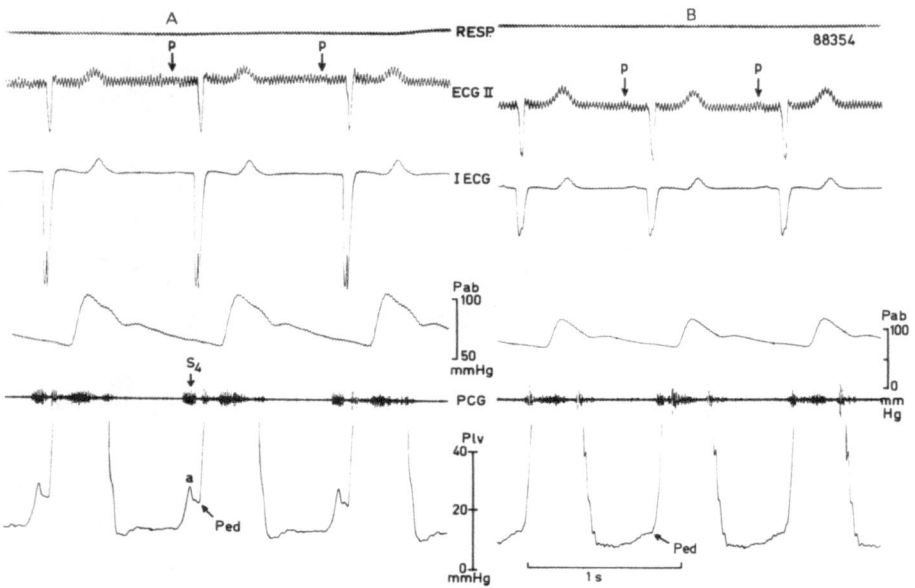

Figure 16. Left atrial activity in hypertrophic cardiomyopathy before (A) and after (B) propranolol.

Hemodynamic data	Panel A	Panel B
Rhythm	NSR	NSR
Heart rate (b/min)	60	73
Ped (mmHg)	22	13
Cardiac output (l/min)	5.2	5.2
Stroke volume (ml)	87	71

Comment: A 43 year old man with non-obstructive hypertrophic cardiomyopathy. Hemodynamic measurements were carried out before (panel A) and after 5 mgr of propranolol intravenously (panel B). The atriogenic pressure rise from 13 to 27 mm of mercury (a, panel A) has completely disappeared after propranolol (panel B) together with the fourth heart sound (S4) in the phonocardiogram (PCG). Despite this loss of mechanical atrial activity, electrical activity is still present as is indicated by the presence of P waves both in the electrocardiogram (ECG) and the intracardiac electrocardiogram (IECG). After propranolol duration of diastole is shortened, heart rate slightly increased while cardiac output remains unchanged. Hence stroke volume decreases from 87 to 71 ml, a loss of 18% of the end-diastolic ventricular volume, which is normal. Transient atrial pump failure was present.

obstruction to outflow is not of major hemodynamic significance to left ventricular function, but the restriction to inflow in combination with left atrial function. (Fig. 17).

The finding of an intraventricular pressure gradient hemodynamically or the observation of a SAM with ASH echocardiographically, though both not specific for HCM, may be useful as diagnostic guides. In this sense, the outflow tract obstruction in HCM still functions as an eyecatcher in attracting the attention for the diagnosis of obstructive (= angulated) HCM.

The severity of the disorder, however, may not be evaluated in my opinion according to the 'severity' of the obstruction expressed either as the degree of narrowing and the duration of mitral-septal contact, or as the labile magnitude of an intraventricular pressure gradient. The severity of the disease is primarily given by the resistance to inflow. Therefore, this might be one of the main reasons for performing a cardiac catheterization in HCM, not in the first place as a diagnostic procedure with measuring an endocavitary pressure gradient, but even more as a research procedure with special attention for measurements of those factors that may be responsible for the severity of ventricular inflow resistance. Furthermore, the influence of pharmacologic agents can be investigated that may give a better insight in the malfunctioning of the individual heart and may permit a better founded conclusion as to the severity of the disease and the potential effect of therapy.

The clinical course of HCM resembles that of a mitral stenosis in several respects if sudden death has not occurred meanwhile. Following the concept of atrioventricle, this is readily understandable with regard to the function of the left atrium. However, in HCM the left atrium is faced with a variable and often progressive hemodynamic resistance and not with a valvular resistance as in mitral stenosis.

In HCM the variable factors that govern the abnormality of filling dynamics, such as cavity size and shape and non-uniformity of myocardial dysfunction, together result in a hemodynamic resistance to ventricular inflow that will have its immediate repercussion on left atrial function. Electrical reactions – such as a spectrum of supraventricular dysrhythmias next to mechanical reactions such as

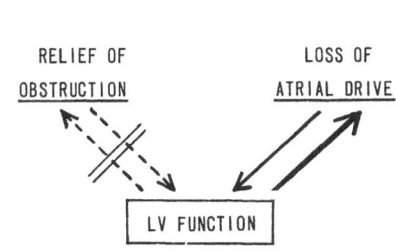

Figure 17. Conceptual triad of hypertrophic cardiomyopathy schematically representing the relevant functional interrelationships in systole and diastole.

hypertrophy and dilatation – may clinically manyfest the left atrial overload. As in mitral stenosis, for instance, atrial fibrillation may occur in long-standing and more advanced cases. There seems to be a certain relationship between the cause of death and the age of the patient, as has been shown by the Bethesda group [3] and by Viersma in our own department [42]. At a mean age of 40 years, congestive heart failure as a 'mechanical' cause of death predominates, whereas the sudden 'electrical' death prevails at a mean age of 19 years.

Within the concept of the atrioventricle it will be apparent that a direct relation exists between the increased left atrial transport function and the decreased left ventricular compliance regardless of the presence or absence of a left ventricular outflow tract obstruction [14]. Hence, the severity, progression and response to treatment may be deduced from signs and symptoms of resistance to ventricular inflow rather than from resistance to ventricular outflow.

The response to *medical* treatment by propranolol and verapamil has already been shown in preceding chapters. Medical treatment of HCM attacks the functional factors that determine obstruction and relaxation (Fig. 18).

Briefly stated here, the negative inotropic and negative chronotropic effects of propranolol may act in reducing the outflow tract gradient by depressing the activity of one or more of the functional factors. However, propranolol (like verapamil) does not have any effect upon the left ventricular end-diastolic compliance (Fig. 19). Clinically, in our experience one of the most important and beneficial effects of propranolol is reducing heart rate, resulting in a lengthening of diastolic filling time and limiting an exercise-induced tachycardia, thereby presumably preventing fatal arrhythmias. However, both propranolol and verapamil [43, 44] do not completely protect against sudden death.

Next to its myocardial depressant effect, verapamil as a calcium antagonist may show a vasodilating effect which in some patients with HCM may result in adverse reactions [45]. Also verapamil in our experiments did not show any influence on the end-diastolic pressure-volume relations (Fig. 20). Bonow et al. [39] could demonstrate in a scintillation study that after verapamil early diastolic filling had improved thereby unloading the left atrium, an 'atrioprotective' effect.

Figure 18. Determinants of obstruction.

A. *Morphologic* factors:
    1. Focal septal deformity above mid-cavity level opposite the AMVL
    2. Presence of AMVL
B. *Functional* factors:
    1. Accelerated blood flow in LVOT due to narrowing
    2. Force, velocity and mode of contraction
    3. Frequency, regularity and mode of electrical activation
    4. Instantaneous volume loading
AMVL: anterior mitral valve leaflet
LVOT: left ventricular outflow tract

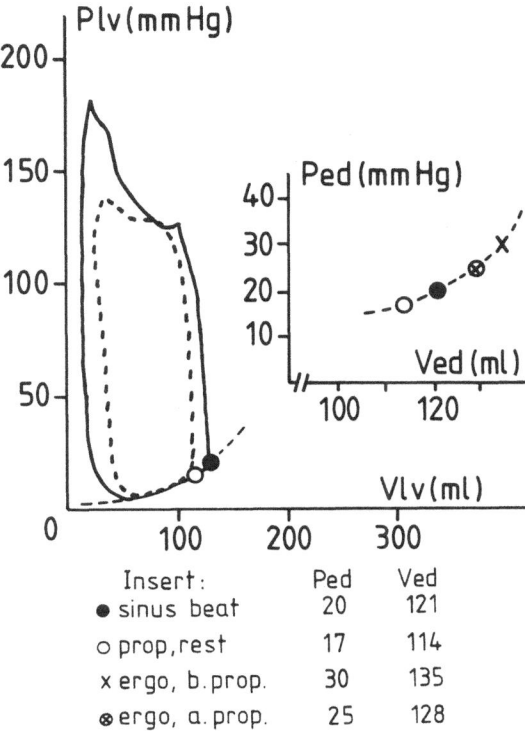

Insert:

	Ped	Ved
● sinus beat	20	121
o prop, rest	17	114
x ergo, b. prop.	30	135
⊗ ergo, a. prop.	25	128

Figure 19. Pressure-volume loops and diastolic pressure-volume relationships in hypertrophic cardio-myopathy at rest and during exercise, before and after propranolol.

A 15 year old boy with obstructive HCM. Drawn line: PV loop during a sinusbeat, before propranolol. Broken line: PV loop during a sinusbeat, after propranolol. After propranolol a decrease in peak-systolic pressure occurs with a diminution in stroke work as manifested by a smaller PV loop.

Insert shows diastolic PV relations at rest (●) and during exercise (x) , and after propranolol (O)(⊗). These different PV relations precisely follow the diastolic compliance curve. No change in end-diastolic compliance occurs after propranolol. So, propranolol may reduce the outflow tract pressure gradient, but leaves the end-diastolic PV relationship unaltered (see also Fig. 4 and Fig. 11).

This 'intradiastolic exchange' of volume of filling may be hypothetically explained by the direct negative inotropic effect of verapamil on the incoordinate relaxation of the ventricular myocardium (Fig. 21).

Non-uniformity of smaller adjacent myocardial areas are thought to be coordinated to a larger more uniformly relaxing area as a result of the depressant action of verapamil mainly effective on the non-affected areas. This 'fusion of non-uniformity' may lead to a less incoordinate relaxation and so might facilitate a greater amount of filling during early diastole.

Clinical experience with *amiodarone* looks very promising especially in cases with serious arrhythmias. Hemodynamic studies with amiodarone have not been done as yet in our laboratory.

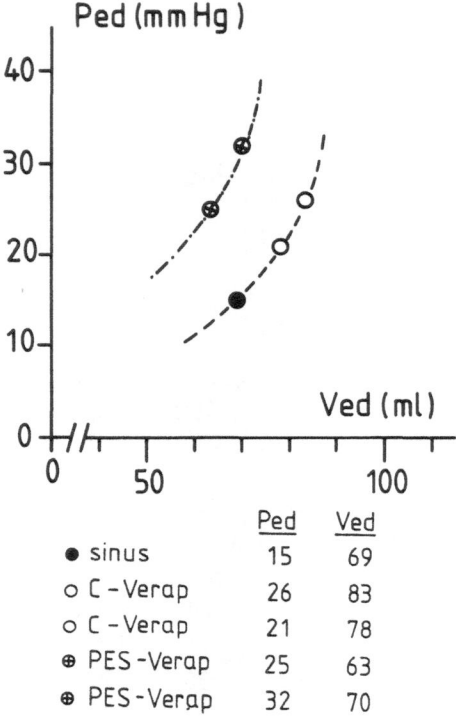

Ped (mmHg)

Ved (ml)

	Ped	Ved
● sinus	15	69
○ C – Verap	26	83
○ C – Verap	21	78
⊕ PES –Verap	25	63
⊕ PES – Verap	32	70

Figure 20. The effect of verapamil on diastolic pressure-volume relationships in hypertrophic cardio-myopathy both at rest and after post-extrasystolic potentiation.

A 56 year old woman with obstructive HCM. C-Verap: on verapamil at rest. PES-Verap: on verapamil after post-extrasystolic potentiation.

This individual example illustrates a shift of the diastolic PV curve leftward and upward indicating further reduction of LV compliance after PES.

Suggested action of Verapamil on improving ventricular relaxation and filling.

FUSION OF NON-UNIFORMITY

– Non-uniformity: area(s) 'out of step'
– Verapamil: N.I. effect, slowing down velocity of relaxation (VR) of 'in step' areas
– Faster VR of 'in step' areas now adapting to slower VR of 'out of step' areas
– Fusion of smaller areas of non-uniformity to a larger area of slowed down uniformity
– Facilitating a larger volume to accommodate in a more uniformly relaxing ventricle.

Surgery is believed to attack primarily the morphologic deformities of outflow tract and ventricular cavity (Fig. 18), thereby providing a remodelling of the outflow tract region and an enlargement of the cavity size [46]. When 'obstruction-minded', one might call this 'relief of obstruction'; when more 'atrium-minded', it represents an increase in ventricular filling capacity.

Like medical treatment, also surgery at any age does not prevent sudden death.

References

1. Rookmaker WA, Nieveen J, Kruizinga K, Blickman JR: Beta-adrenergic blockade in the treatment of left-sided hypertrophic obstructive cardiomyopathy (HOCM). Acta Med Scand 189:427–431, 1971.
2. Frank S, Braunwald E: Idiopathic hypertrophic subaortic stenosis. Clinical analysis of 126 patients with emphasis on the natural history. Circulation 37:759–788, 1968.
3. Maron BJ, Lipson LC, Roberts WC, Savage DD, Epstein SE: Malignant hypertrophic cardiomyopthy: identification of a subgroup of families with unusually frequent premature death. Am J Cardiol 41:1133–1140, 1978.
4. McKenna WJ, England D, Doi L, Deanfield JE, Oakley CM, Goodwin JF: Arrhythmias in hypertrophic cardiomyopathy. I. Influence on prognosis. Brit Heart J 46:168–172, 1981.
5. Goodwin JF: The frontiers of cardiomyopathy. Brit Heart J 118:1–18, 1982.
6. Beahrs MM, Tajik AJ, Seward JB, Giuliani ER, McGoon DC: Hypertrophic Obstructive Cardiomyopathy: ten- to 21-year follow-up after partial septal myectomy. Am J Cardiol 51:1160–1166, 1983.
7. Maron BJ, Roberts WC, Epstein SE: Sudden death in hypertrophic cardiomyopathy: a profile of 78 patients. Circulation 65:1388–1394, 1982.
8. Hernandez RR, Greenfield JC, McCall BW: Pressure-flow studies in hypertrophic subaortic stenosis. J Clin Invest 43:401–407, 1964.
9. Pierce GE, Morrow AG, Braunwald E: Idiopathic hypertrophic subaortic stenosis. III. Intraoperative studies of the mechanism of obstruction and its hemodynamic consequences. Circulation 30 (suppl. 4): 152–213, 1964.
10. Ross Jr J, Braunwald E, Gault JH, Mason DT, Morrow AG: The mechanism of the intraventricular pressure gradient in idiopathic hypertrophic subaortic stenosis. Circulation 34:558–578, 1966.
11. Van der Wall E: Hypertrophic obstructive cardiomyopathy. Evaluation of treatment by invasive and non-invasive methods. Thesis, Groningen, 1972.
12. Van der Wall E: Hypertrophic obstructive cardiomyopathy. Evaluation of left ventricular function by non-invasive methods. Neth J Med 17:157, 1974.
13. Van der Wall E: Hypertrofische obstructieve cardiomyopathie. De amylnitriet provocatietest als middel tot evaluatie van therapie. (Amylnitrite provocation test as on aid to evaluation of therapy in HOCM). Hart Bulletin 6:60–66, 1975.
14. Van der Wall E, Bergstra A, Blickman JR, Kruizinga K, Kuipers JRG, Mook GA: Left atrial activity in hypertrophic cardiomyopathy. Hemodynamic and angiocardiographic aspects. 7th Eur Congress of Cardiol, abstract book I, 1976, p 592.
15. Van der Wall E, Mook GA: Exercise and atrial pacing in hypertrophic cardiomyopathy before and after administration of propranolol. VIIIth world congress Cardiol, abstract, Tokio, 1978.
16. Henry WL, Clark CE, Epstein SE: Asymmetric septal hypertrophy (ASH): echocardiographic identification of the pathognomonic anatomic abnormality of IHSS. Circulation 47:225–233, 1973.

17. Henry WL, Clark CE, Griffith JM, Epstein SE: Mechanism of left ventricular outflow obstruction in patients with obstructive asymmetric septal hypertrophy (idiopathic hypertrophic subaortic stenosis). Am J Cardiol 35:337–345, 1975.
18. Maron BJ, Roberts WG: Quantitative analysis of cardiac muscle cell disorganization in the ventricular septum in patients with hypertrophic cardiomyopathy. Circulation 59:689–706, 1979.
19. Maron BJ, Epstein SE: Hypertrophic cardiomyopathy. Recent observations regarding the specificity of three hallmarks of the disease: asymmetric septal hypertrophy, septal cell disorganization and systolic anterior motion of the anterior mitral leaflet. Am J Cardiol 45:141–154, 1980.
20. Maron BJ, Gottdiener KS, Epstein SE: Patterns and significance of distribution of left ventricular hypertrophy in hypertrophic cardiomyopathy. A wide-angle, two-dimensional echocardiographic study of 125 patients. Am J Cardiol 48:418–428, 1981.
21. Bulkley BH, Weisfeldt ML, Hutchins GM: Asymmetric septal hypertrophy and myocardial fiber disarray. Features of normal, developing and malformed hearts. Circulation 56:292–298, 1977.
22. Maron BJ, Verter J, Kapur S: Disproportionate ventricular septal thickening in the developing normal human heart. Circulation 57:520–526, 1978.
23. Teare D: Asymmetrical hypertrophy of the heart in young patients. Brit Heart J 20:1–8, 1958.
24. Falicov RE, Resnekow L: Mid-ventricular obstruction in hypertrophic obstructive cardiomyopathy. New diagnostic and therapeutic challenge. Brit Heart J 39:701–705, 1977.
25. Yamaguchi H, Ishimura T, Nishiyama S, Nagasaki F, Nakanishi S, Takatsu f, Nishijo T, Umeda T, Machii K: Hypertrophic non-obstructive cardiomyopathy with giant negative T waves (apical hypertrophy): ventriculographic and echocardiographic features in 30 patients. Am J Cardiol 44: 401–412, 1979.
26. Spirito P, Maron BJ: Significance of left ventricular outflow tract cross-sectional area in hypertrophic cardiomyopathy: a two-dimensional echocardiographic assessment. Circulation 67:1100-1108, 1983.
27. St. John Sutton MG, Tajik AJ, Smith HC, Ritman EL: Angina in idiopathic hypertrophic stenosis. A clinical correlate of regional left ventricular dysfunction: a videometric and echocardiographic study. Circulation 61:561–568, 1980.
28. Sanderson JE, Gibson DG, Brown DJ, Goodwin JF: Left ventricular filling in hypertrophic cardiomyopathy. An angiographic study. Brit Heart J 39:661–670, 1977.
29. Pollick Ch, Morgan Ch, Gilbert B, Rakowski H, Wigle ED: The relation between SAM and the pressure gradient in muscular subaortic stenosis. Circulation 60 (suppl II):606, 1979.
30. Wilson WS, Criley JM, Ross RS: Dynamics of left ventricular emptying in hypertrophic subaortic stenosis: a cineangiographic and hemodynamic study. Am Heart J 73:4–16, 1967.
31. Murgo JP, Alter BR, Dorethy JF, Altobelli SA, McGrananhan GM: Dynamics of left ventricular ejection in obstructive and non-obstructive hypertrophic cardiomyopathy. J Clin Invest 66:1369–1382, 1980.
32. Murgo JP, Alter BR, Dorethy JF, Altobelli SA, Craig WE, McGranahan GM: The effects of intraventricular gradients on left ventricular ejection dynamics. Eur Heart J 4 (suppl F):23–28, 1983.
33. Goodwin JF: Hypertrophic cardiomyopathy: a disease in search of its own identity. Am J Cardiol 45:177–180, 1980.
34. Ruskin J, McHale PA, Harley A, Greenfield JC: Pressure-flow studies in man: effects of atrial systole on left ventricular function. J Clin Invest 49: 472–478, 1970.
35. Hammermeister KE, Warbasse JR: The rate of change of left ventricular volume in man. II. Diastolic events in health and disease. Circulation 49:739–747, 1974.
36. Silver MA, Bonow RO, Deglin SM, Cannon RO, Roberts WC: Acquired left ventricular endocardial constriction from massive calcific deposits: a newly recognized cause of impairment to left ventricular filling. Am J Cardiol 53:1468–1470, 1984.
37. Blanksma PK: Pressure-volume and stress-strain relationships in hypertrophic cardiomyopathy (HCM). In: Van der Wall E, Lie KI (eds), Recent views on hypertrophic cardiomyopathy. Martinus Nijhoff, Dordrecht, 1985, pp 53–69.

38. Bonow RO, Frederick TM, Bacharach SL, Green MV, Goose PW, Maron BJ, Rosing DR: Atrial systole and left ventricular filling in hypertrophic cardiomyopathy: effect of verapamil. Am J Cardiol 51:1386–1391, 1983.

39. Bonow RO, Ostrow HG, Rosing DR, Cannon III RO, Lipson LC, Maron BJ, Kent KM, Bacharach SL, Green MV: Effects of verapamil on left ventricular systolic and diastolic function in patients with hypertrophic cardiomyopathy: pressure-volume analysis with a non-imaging scintillation probe. Circulation 68:1062–1073, 1983.

40. Ten Cate FJ, Serruys PW, Mey S, Roelandt J: Effects of short-term administration of verapamil on left ventricular relaxation and filling dynamics measured by a combined hemodynamic – ultrasonic technique in patients with hypertrophic cardiomyopathy. Circulation 68:1274–1279, 1983.

41. Hanrath P, Schlüter M, Sonntag F, Diemert J, Bleifeld W: Influence of verapamil therapy at rest and during exercise in hypertrophic cardiomyopathy. Am J Cardiol 52: 544–548, 1983.

42. Viersma JW, Postma DS, Van Veldhuizen DJ, Hamer JPM, Postma DS, Van der Wall E: Arrhythmias in hypertrophic cardiomyopathy: prognostic significance and clinical relevance. In: Van der Wall E, Lie KI (eds), Recent views on hypertrophic cardiomyopathy. Martinus Nijhoff, Dordrecht, 1985, pp 21–31.

43. Kaltenbach M: Treatment of hypertrophic obstructive cardiomyopathy with verapamil. Brit Heart J 42:35–42.

44. Hopf R, Kaltenbach M: Verapamil treatment of hypertrophic cardiomyopathy. In: Kaltenbach M, Epstein SE (eds), Hypertrophic cardiomyopathy; the therapeutic role of calcium antagonists. Springer, Berlin, 1982, pp 163–178.

45. Epstein SE, Rosing DR: Verapamil: its potential for causing serious complications in patients with hypertrophic cardiomyopathy. Circulation 64: 437–441, 1981.

46. Reis RL, Hannah III H, Carley JE, Pugh DM: Surgical treatment of idiopathic hypertrophic subaortic stenosis (IHSS): postoperative results in 30 patients following ventricular septal myotomy and myectomy (Morrow procedure). Circulation 56 (suppl II, no 3):128–132, 1977.

7. Treatment of hypertrophic cardiomyopathy with beta blockers or calcium antagonists

M. KALTENBACH and R. HOPF

Abstract. Sixty-one consecutive patients with well-defined hypertrohic cardiomyopathy were treated with calcium channel blockers (60 patients with verapamil at average dose 530 mg (320–720 mg/d) and one patient received 30 mg nifedipine). All patients had clinical, non-invasive and cardiac catheterization evaluation at the time of entry into the study. Therapy was continued for an average of 54 months (10–98). Follow-up studies were systematically performed at 6 month intervals.

Subjective improvement was achieved in 47 out of 55 symptomatic patients (85%). Heart size, judged as heart volume from telechest-X-ray in supine position, showed a reduction in 36/61, no change in 15/61 and in 10/61 was increased. On average in all 61 patients, a significant reduction from 947 to 833 ml/1.73 m² was seen. Twenty-six patients who had been followed for an average of 24 months prior to verapamil therapy on beta blockers or no treatment had heart volume increases averaging 12% in the preverapamil treatment.

The ECG showed a significant reduction in QRS amplitude and a tendency towards normalization of ST/T segments. Serial echocardiography study showed small but significant reduction in septal and free wall thickness as well as in left atrial diameter. Repeat catheterization was performed in 19 patients and a significant reduction in intraventricular pressure gradient, left ventricular muscle mass and coronary artery diameter was demonstrated.

Three patients died during the study (256 patient-treatment-years) for an annual mortality rate of 1.3%. This mortality is considerably lower than reported for patients receiving no treatment, beta blockade, or surgery. In the entire series only one patient had surgery related to the hypertrophic cardiomyopathy and only one patient had verapamil dose reduced because of the occurrence of heart block. No patient discontinued the drug because of side-effects.

Utilizing serial non-invasive and invasive studies, we conclude that verapamil therapy in hypertrophic cardiomyopathy results in objective and subjective improvement, a low death rate and a low incidence of operation as compared to standard therapy.

Hypertrophic cardiomyopathy (HCM) has been described by more than 50 terms since the original description by Schmincke in 1907 [1].

The entity is characterized by:
- left, and occasionally right, ventricular hypertrophy without ventricular dilatation;
- normal to hypernormal left ventricular systolic function;
- diastolic dysfunction with impaired left ventricular filling characteristics;
- and the presence of left ventricular outflow tract obstruction in some patients.

The presice histologic picture in HCM is controversial. When compared to the dilated forms of cardiomyopathy, the total muscle mass is often less in HCM. Kunkel et al. [2] have shown that the increase in myocardial fiber diameter is more pronounced in dilated cardiomyopathy than in HCM.

The functional characteristics of cardiomyopathy, especially in its early stages, suggest increased sympathetic stimulation. However, increased beta-sympathetic activity does not explain the syndrome since patients with the hyperkinetic heart syndrome [3] have well documented increased sympathetic activity and hypernormal cardiac function but do not undergo hypertrophy. In addition, the hyperkinetic heart syndrome is treated effectively with beta blockers while hypertrophic cardiomyopathy has generally shown disappointing response to longterm therapy [5].

Hypertrophic cardiomyopathy has features suggesting intracellular calcium overload with increased intracellular calcium-ion-availability. The effect of digitalis in producing an increased intraventricular gradient tends to support this hypothesis [4]. Hence, assuming that calcium ions play a role in the evolution and manifestation of hypertrophic cardiomyopathy, therapy with calcium channel blockers seems rational. We initiated a study utilizing calcium channel blockers in 1973. Preliminary reports were made, starting in 1976 [6–8]. The current report is the longterm follow-up of our experience.

Patients and methods

Sixty-one consecutive patients were entered into the study. In every patient the diagnosis was established by clinical findings, M-mode and 2D-echograms, and left and right heart catheterization with ventriculography and selective coronary arteriography. Forty-four patients had left intraventricular pressure gradients between 32 and 290 mmHg (average 99 mmHg) at rest or with provocative manoeuvres. In 17 patients the gradient was 30 mmHg or less at rest or following provocation. No patient with HCM was excluded from the study because of the severity of his/her disease. During the entire study, only four patients interrupted verapamil therapy. The reasons included a severe automobil accident, non-cardiac surgery, intercurrent disease, and an unwillingnes to continue the drug. In three patients, verapamil therapy was resumed after an interval of 6–15 months. Surgery related to the cardiomyopathy was performed in only one instance.

All medications were discontinued before the institution of calcium channel blocker therapy. The orally administered verapamil dose averaged 530 mg (320–720 mg/d). One patient was treated with nifedipine 30 mg/d. Patients experiencing severe arrhythmias after instituting verapamil therapy were given additional antiarrhythmic drugs such as ajmaline bitartrate, and in one patient, amiodarone. The mean duration of therapy was 54 months (10–96). Twenty-two patients were treated for more than 5 years. The total experience respresents 256 patient-treatment-years. Patients were followed closely during the first 3 months. Thereafter, they were seen every 6–12 months and physical examination, ECG, carotid pulse, echocardiogram, chest-X-ray and heart volume determination (calculated from tele-chest-X-rays in supine position) were repeated. In all patients verapamil plasma levels were determined and served as a guide to dose adjustment.

Repeat cardiac catheterization was performed 19 patients at an average of 26 months following the institution of therapy (8–52 months).

Results

In 47 out of 55 patients (85%) the symptoms had improved or disappeared during verapamil therapy. Symptoms were unchanged in seven patients (11%) and worsened in one patient. Six patients were free of complaints prior to therapy and remained so during treatment. Utilizing New York Heart Association classification, there was an improvement from class 2.7 to 1.9 when all 61 patients are included (Fig. 1).

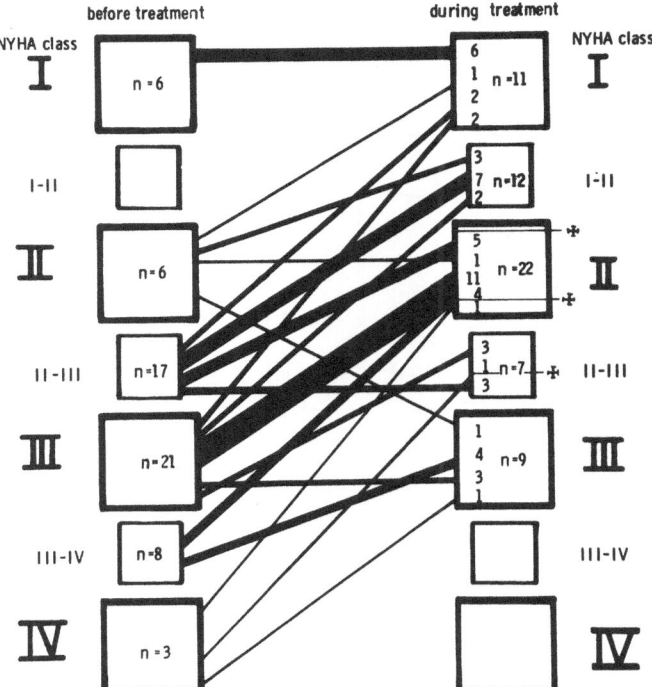

Figure 1. Improvement in symptoms according to NYH classification.

Among specific complaints the improvement in exertional dyspnea and angina was most impressive. Episodes of syncope and/or collapse improved or disappeared in all patients who presented with this symptom. The subjective improvement noted by patients was confirmed by improved exercise tolerance on objective testing.

Electrocardiogram

Serial electrocardiographic studies were utilized to follow left ventricular hypertrophy. R and S amplitude were carefully measured in the precordial leads. In a subgroup of 39 patients, serial ECGs prior to the institution of verapamil therapy showed an increase from 4.64 to 4.99 mV in the QRS amplitude. For the entire 61 patients during verapamil therapy, a decrease in QRS amplitude occurred, averaging 4.82 to 4.37 mV. Thirty-six patients showed a decrease in QRS amplitude, 13 remained unchanged and 12 increased. ST/T changes were not studied in a quantitative fashion, but improvement in ST/T abnormalities tended to parallel reduction in QRS amplitude. However, return of the ECG to a normal parameter was seen in only a rare patient (Figs. 2, 3).

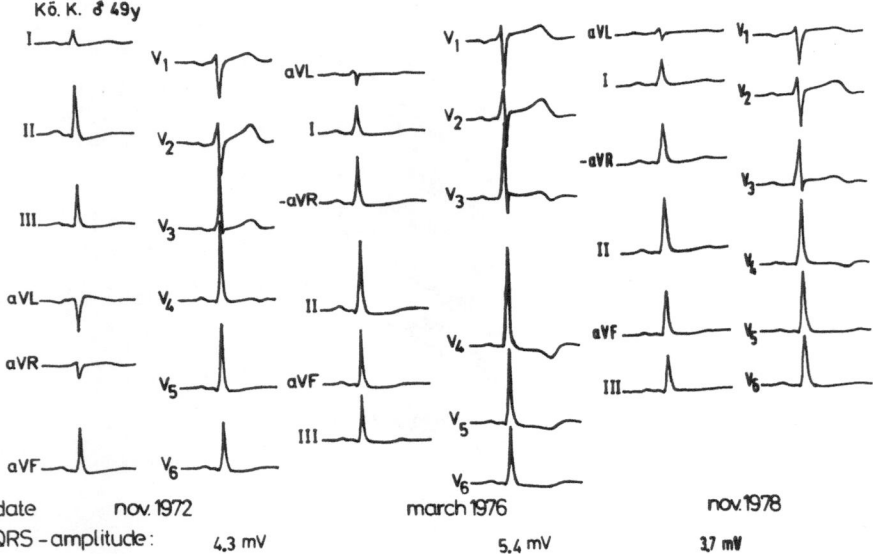

Figure 2. ECG of a 49 year old man with HCM. Deterioration can be seen after 4 years with beta blocker treatment. After 2 years verapamil treatment QRS amplitude decreased and ST-T changes were slightly improved.

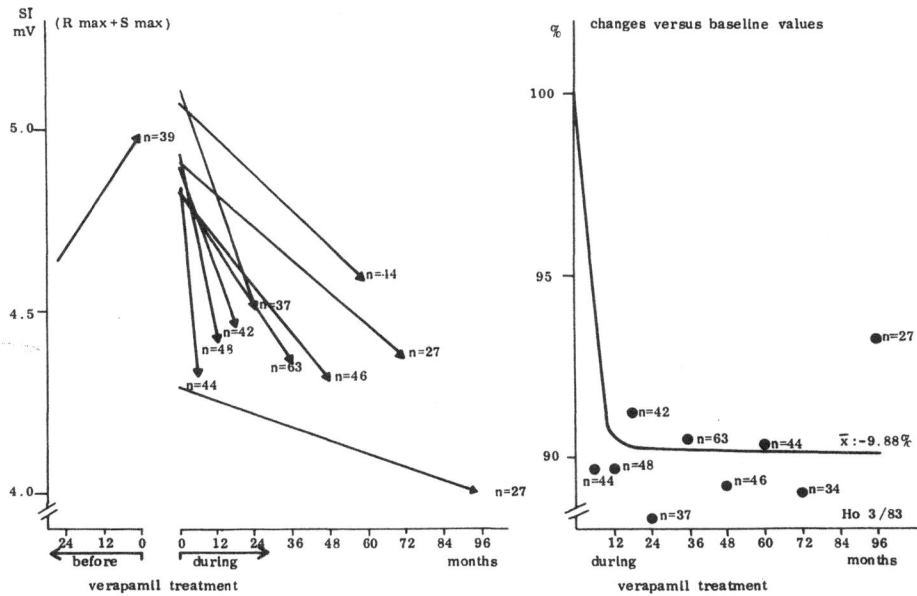

Figure 3. Increase of QRS amplitude during pre-treatment period and decrease during verapamil treatment.

Carotid pulse, phonogram

From the patients with the obstuctive form of the disease and a typical pulse with systolic double impulse 30% showed complete normalization of the tracings during therapy. Figure 4 gives an example. The systolic murmur remained generally unchanged.

Chest-X-ray

Cardiac figuration on chest-X-ray performed in a standing position remained unchanged during treatment. In no instance did new signs of pulmonary congestion or deterioration of pre-existing congestion occur during verapamil therapy. Heart volume determinations from the supine chest-X-ray were performed by serial study in 26 patients prior to the institution of verapamil therapy. The average interval between the studies was 26 months. The mean value before beta blocker therapy was 871 ml/1.73 m² and increased during beta blockade further by 11% (from 871 to 975 ml/1.73 m²); the normal range for male is 620 ± 170, for female 570 ± 120 ml/1.73 m² (x ± 25).

During verapamil therapy supine heart volume determinations were made

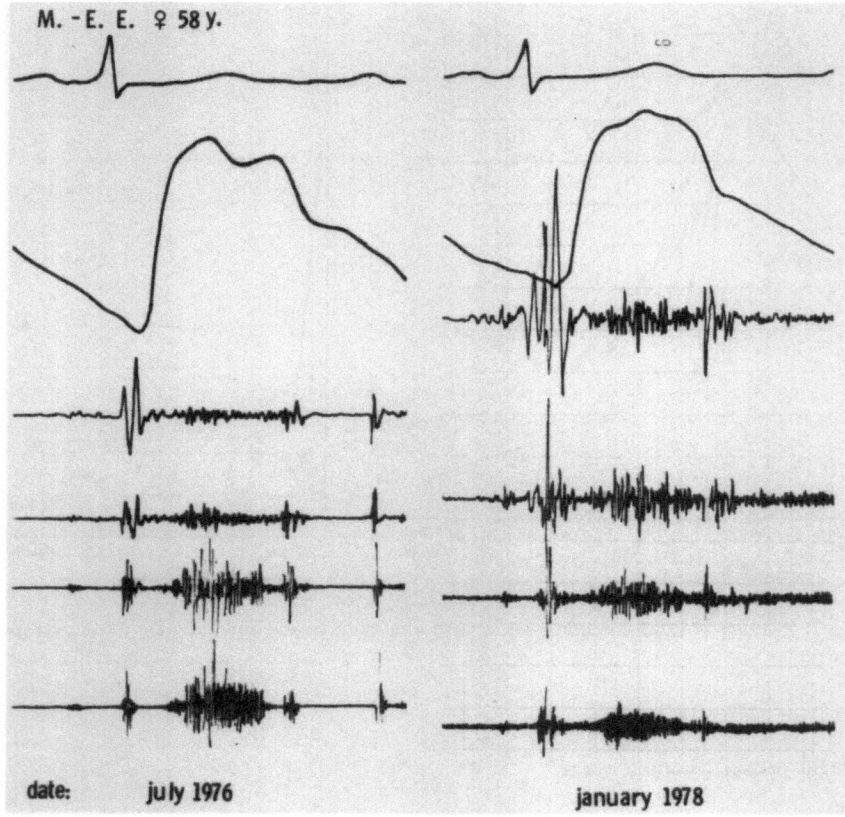

M. - E. E. ♀ 58 y.

date: july 1976   january 1978

Figure 4. Normalization of carotid pulse during verapamil treatment.

serially in all 61 patients, volume decreased by 9% (912 to 833 ml/1.73 m²). Thirty-six patients had a decreased heart volume, 15 showed no change and 10 had an increase. Of the 22 patients followed for more than 5 years, no patient had an increase in heart size during longterm observation (Figs. 5, 6).

Echocardiogram

The echocardiograms performed on entry to the study showed the left ventricular cavity to be normal (≤5.5 cm) in all patients. Septal wall thickness and/or free wall thickness was increased (≥1.3 cm). Eighty percent of the patients had left atrial diameters exceeding 5 cm.

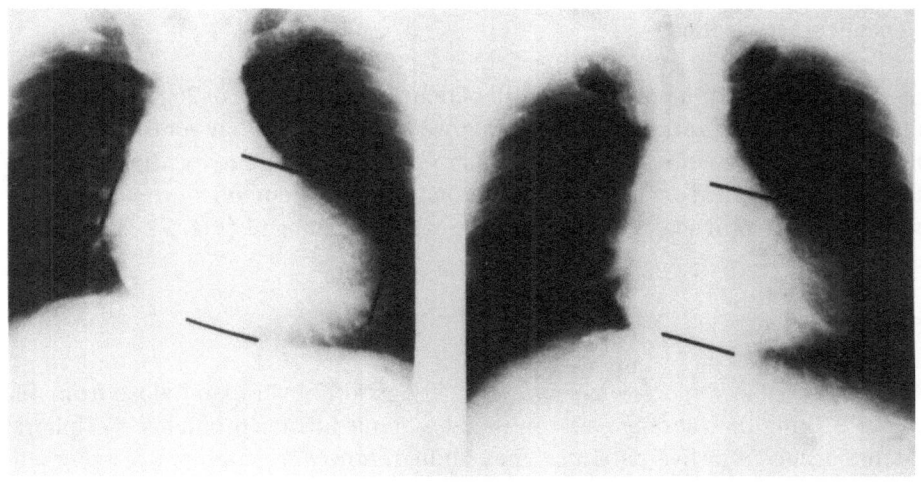

Figure 5. Example of heart volume normalization during verapamil treatment. Only the p.a. chest-X-ray is shown (supine position); left side before, right side after 3 years verapamil treatment.

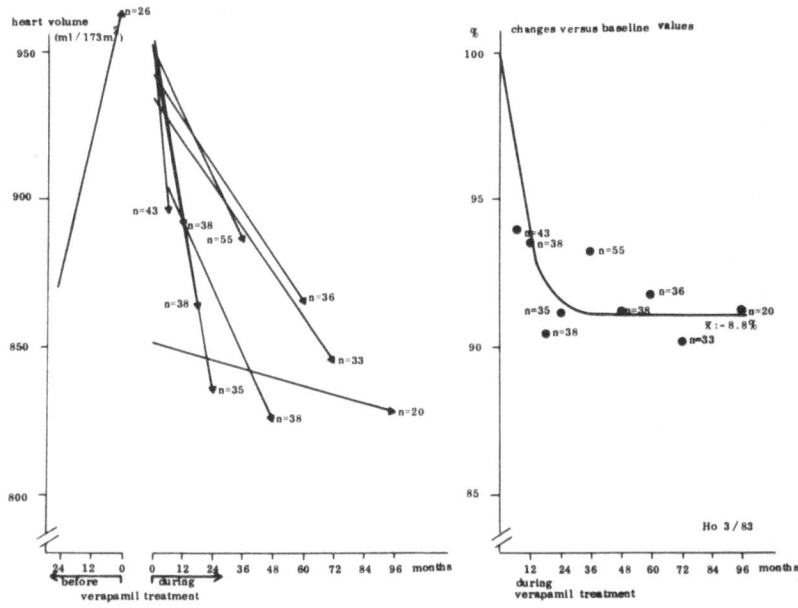

Figure 6. Increase in heart volume during pre-treatment period and decrease during verapamil treatment.

Repeat catheterization

Serial catheterization performed in 19 patients at an interval of 26 (8–52) months after institution of verapamil therapy showed no change in left ventricular systolic and diastolic volumes. Left ventricular gradient during provocation, left ventricular muslce mass and the average coronary artery diameter were significantly reduced. Left ventricular filling pressure was not changed (Fig. 7).

Side effects

In one patient AV-block was seen. After reduction of verapamil dose from 480 mg to 320 mg the therapy was continued without further problems. Peripheral edema occurred in five patients. They all had, however, some pre-existing tendency to peripheral fluid retention. Symptoms were controlled by diuretics. Other side effects were increased diaphoresis, headache, vertigo and constipation. These complaints usually improved or disappeared with longterm medication; constipation, however, sometimes required laxatives. No serious side effects such as pulmonary edema or heart failure were observed.

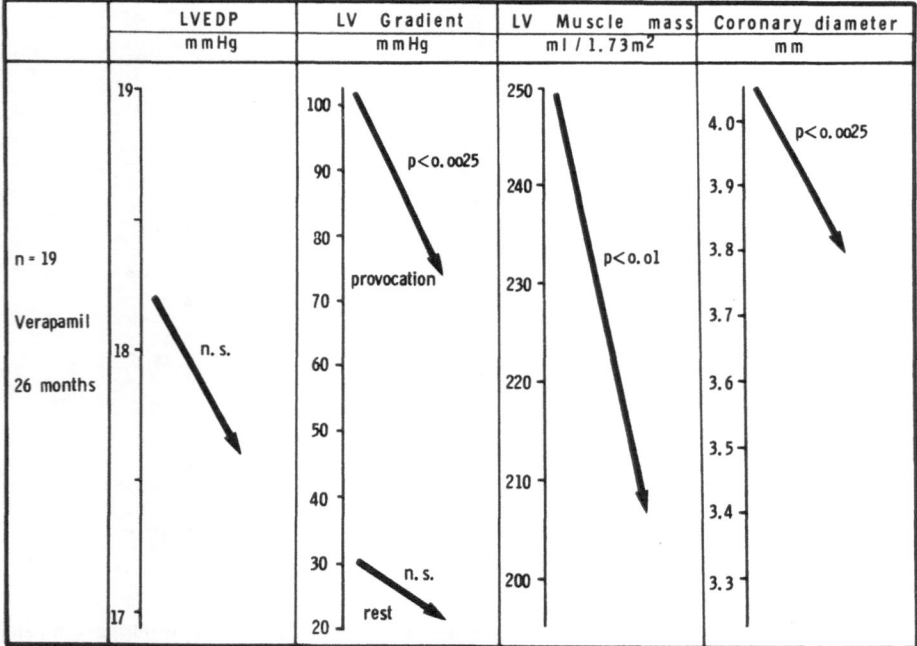

Figure 7. Hemodynamics, left ventricular muscle mass and coronary artery diameters from 19 patients recatheterized after 26 months of verapamil treatment.

Operation

Only one patient included in the study had heart surgery related to the disease. This patient had shown slow clinical deterioration during a preceding treatment period with 480 mg propranolol/day. After initiation of verapamil treatment his symptoms slightly improved, heart volume decreased. However, he continued to have episodes of dyspnea and pulmonary congestion. When he was first seen the left intraventricular pressure gradient at rest was 36, during provocation 64 mmHg. After 3 years propranolol treatment recatheterization revealed a gradient of 88 at rest and 160 after provocation; LVEDP had increased from 18 to 29 mmHg. After 1½ year of verapamil treatment despite subjective improvement the gradient had further increased to 116 at rest and 184 after provocation, while LVEDP had decreased to 11 mmHg (Table 1). In this situation septal myec tomy was successfully performed (Prof. Bircks, Düsseldorf, FRH). After operation verapamil therapy was continued.

Mortality

During the treatment period of 10–96 months (average 54 months) three patients died, two on verapamil, one on nifedipine. In two patients sudden death occurred, one patient with the non-obstructive form died in cardiogenic shock. Mortality rate calculated from the 61 patients treated over an average of 54 months, i.e. 256 patient-treatment-years, was 3/256 or 1.3%.

Table 1. Invasive and non-invasive findings of a patient who was operated because his symptoms were not sufficiently controlled during verapamil treatment. During 3 years of preceding propranolol therapy all parameters had deteriorated, during verapamil therapy left ventricular filling pressure and heart volume decreased but the gradient increased further.

	Propranolol	Verapamil	
Left heart catheterization	May 78	Febr. 81	April 83
LV gradient (mmHg rest-prov.)	36 - 64	88 - 160	116 - 184
LVEDP (mmHg)	18	29	11
QRS amplitude (cm)	5.5	5.6	5.2
Heart volume ml/1.73 m²)	1010	1240	1135
Echo: LA (cm)	5.1	5.4	5.3
IVS (cm)	–	2.9	2.9
PLVW (cm)	–	1.9	1.8

Discussion

Patients with hypertrophic cardiomyopathy show a highly variable course ranging from asymptomatic forms with a normal life expectancy to patients who die suddenly at early adult age or even during childhood. Treatment with beta blockers has been applied for more than 20 years but no substantial longterm benefit has been demonstrated [5, 9]. Surgery generally shows impressive hemodynamic improvement, however, there is no evidence of improved longevity. Recidivations after successful surgery have been reported and transition to the dilated form of cardiomyopathy seems to occur [10–12].

Therapy with calcium channel blockers appears a rational form of treatment

(a) from theoretical reasons: Ca-ion overload may have an etiological role or may be an important part of the vicious circle leading to the different manifestations of HCM;

(b) from clinical reasons: Calcium channel blockers enhance ventricular relaxation. Diastolic abnormality, i.e. increased ventricular stiffness, is an important pathophysiologic feature of the disease. Some calcium channel blockers, in particularly verapamil, have also an effect on systolic function with a slight negative influence on systolic ventricular performance. In contrast to beta blockade this effect can be easily overcome by increased sympathetic stimuli.

We report a large experience with 61 consecutive patients followed over 256 patients-years including 22 patients for more than 5 years.

The most impressive clinical observation is subjective improvement in symptoms such as exertional angina and dyspnea. Patients pretreated with beta blockers often report less side effects such as general fatigue and impotence. The increased working capacity can be documented by exercise testing. Objective findings from serial ECG and echocardiography showed slight reduction in left ventricular hypertrophy. Serial heart volume determination has revealed in the whole treatment group a reduction in heart size. Some patients returned into the normal range of heart volume and patients treated over more than 5 years showed no late increase.

Serial heart catheterization performed in 19 patients showed in no case transition to the dilated form of cardiomyopathy. Left ventricular volumes remained within the normal range.

Left ventricular gradient and left ventricular muscle mass were slightly reduced. The reduction in average coronary artery diameter is probably the consequence of reduced hypertrophy resulting in a reduced myocardial muscle mass. From clinical and pathological studies a positive relationship is known between degree of ventricular hypertrophy and average coronary artery diameter [13].

Survival rate can apparently only be determined from very large series since the

Table 2. Longterm mortality in patients with no treatment, propranolol or operation according to different authors.

	Treatment				
	No	Propranolol 120-240 MG	Operation	Operation	Operation
Patient-years	315	362	660	1165	468
Mort/year.*	3.4%	2.8%	3.0%	3.7%	3.3%
Authors	Loogen, Kuhn 1976 [9]	Kuhn, Loogen 1978 [5]	Rothlin, Senning 1976	Maron, Epstein 1978 [10]	Beahrs, McGoon 1983 [12]

* General average 3.24%

reported mortality rate is only about 3% per year. From the literature an average value of 3.3% ranging from 2.8 to 3.7 can be calculated derived from a total of 2970 patient-years (Table 2). Derived from the observation of 256 patient-years during verapamil treatment a rate of 1.3% was calculated. It can be concluded that death rate is certainly not deteriorated by this treatment and may possibly be improved as compared to patients receiving beta blockers, surgery or no treatment. The favorable results with verapamil treatment have been confirmed by several authors [14–21].

Thus, from a pathophysiological point of view as well as from clinical experience the therapy of hypertrophic cardiomyopathy with calcium channel blockers appears to be the preferred form of drug therapy. In contrast to beta blockade calcium channel blockers improve left ventricular filling characteristics which often play a dominant role in the manifestation of the disease [22–24].

The favorable influence on diastolic ventricular performance appears to occur after different calcium channel blockers, however, the influence on systolic function cannot be documented after nifedipine (except intracoronary application). Verapamil exhibits slight negative inotropic effects after intravenous as well as after oral application. Therefore, this type of calcium blockers may be superior to other drugs in the therapy of hypertrophic cardiomyopathy [25, 26].

Acknowledgement. The autors are most indebted to G.C. Friesinger, M.D., Nashville, U.S.A., for his critics and his help to finish this manuscript.

References

1. Schmincke A: Über linksseitige muskuläre Conusstenosen. Dtsch Med Wschr 33:1082, 1907.

112

2. Kunkel B, Schneider M, Hopf R, Kober G, Hübner K, Kaltenbach M: Left ventricular biopsy in hypertrophic cardiomyopathy: light and electron microscopic evaluations.
3. Gorlin R: The hyperkinetic heart syndrome. J Am Med Ass 182:823–929, 1962.
4. Fleckenstein A: Calcium-antagonism in heart and smooth muscle. John Whiley, New York, 1983.
5. Kuhn H, Loogen F: Die Anwendung von Beta-Rezeptorenblockern bei hypertrophischer obstruktiver Kardiomyopathie. Internist 19:527, 1978.
6. Kaltenbach M, Hopf R, Keller M: Calcium-antagonistische Therapie bei hypertrophischer obstruktiver Kardiomyopathie. Dtsch Med Wschr 101:1284, 1976.
7. Kaltenbach M, Hopf R, Kober G, Bussmann W-D, Keller M, Petersen Y: Treatment of hypertrophic obstructive cardiomyopathy with Verapamil. Brit Heart J 42:35, 1979.
8. Kaltenbach M, Epstein S-E (eds): Hypertrophic Cardiomyopathy. Springer, Berlin, 1982.
9. Loogen F, Krelhaus W, Kuhn H: Verlaufsbeobachtungen der hypertrophischen obstruktiven Kardiomyopathie (HOCM). Z Kardiol 65:511, 1976.
10. Maron BJ, Merill WH, Freier PA, Kent KM, Epstein SE, Morrow AG: Longterm clinical course and symptomatic status of patients after operation for hypertrophic subaortic stenosis. Circulation 57:1205, 1978.
11. Rothlin M, Arbenz N, Krayenbühl HP Turina J Senning A: Spätresultate nach Operationen bei muskulärer subvalvulärer Aortenstenose. Z Kardiol 65:501, 1976.
12. Beahrs MM, Tajik AJ, Seward JB, Giuliani EJ, McGoon DC: Hypertrophic obstructive cardiomyopathy: 10 to 21-year follow-up after partial septal myectomy. Am J Cardiol 51:1160–1166, 1983.
13. Kober G, Spahn G, Becker H-J, Kaltenbach M: Weite und Querschnittsfläche der Großen epikardialen Koronararterien bei Herzmuskelhypertrophie. Z Kardiol 63:297, 1973.
14. Troesch M, Hirzel HO, Jenni R, Krayenbühl HP: Langzeittherapie mit Verapamil bei hypertrophischer Kardiomyopathie. Schweiz Med Wschr 109:1683, 1979.
15. Rosing DR, Kent KM, Maron BJ, Epstein SE: Verapamil therapy: a new approach to the pharmacologic treatment of hypertrophic cardiomyopathy. II. Effects on exercise capacity and symptomatic status. Circulation 60:1208–1213, 1979.
16. Schmidt P, Pavek P, Klein W: Echokardiographische und hämodynamische Untersuchungen zur Beeinflussung der hypertrophischen obstruktiven Kardiomyopathie durch Verapamil. Z Kardiol 68:89–92, 1979.
17. Rosing DR, Kent KM, Borer HS, Seides SF, Maron BJ, Epstein SE: Verapamil therapy: a new approach to the pharmacologic treatment of hypertrophic cardiomyopathy. I. hemodynamic effects. Circulation 60:1201–1207, 1979.
18. Bonow RO, Rosing DR, Bacharach SL, Green MV, Lipson LC, Condit JR, Kent KM, Epstein SE: Longterm effects of verapamil on left ventricular diastolic filling in patients with hypertrophic cardiomyopathy. Am J Cardiol 47:409, 1981.
19. Kober G, Hopf R, Schmidt A, Kaltenbach M, Biamino G, Schröder R, Bubenheimer P, Roskamm H, Hanrath P, Sonntag F, v. Olshausen K, Zebe H, Kübler W, Schönung W, Müller A, Schlepper M: Longterm treatment of hypertrophic cardiomyopathy with verapamil or propranolol. Preliminary results of a multicenter study. 8:261–269.
20. Haberer T, Hess OM, Jenni R, Krayenbühl HP: Hypertrophic obstructive cardiomyopathy: spontaneous course in comparison to longterm therapy with propranolol and verapamil. Z Kardiol 72:487–493, 1983.
21. Raff GL, Brundage BH, Ports TA, Chatterjee K: Dissociation between acute hemodynamic effects and clinical response to verapamil in hypertrophic cardiomyopathy. Clin Res 29:79A, 1981.
22. Hanrath P, Mathey DG, Vremer P, Sonntag F, Bleifeld W: Effect of verapamil on left ventricular isovolumic relaxation time and regional left ventricular filling in hypertrophic cardiomyopathy. Am J Cardiol 45:1258, 1979.

23. Lorell BH, Paulus WJ, Grossmann W, Wynne J, Cohn PF, Braunwald E: Improved diastolic function and systolic performance in hypertrophic cardiomyopathy after nifedipine. N Engl J Med 303:801, 1980.

24. Bonow RO, Ostrow HG, Rosing DR, Cannon III RO, Lipson LC, Maron BJ, Kent KM, Bacharach SL, Green MV: Effects of verapamil on left ventricular systolic and diastolic function in patients with hypertrophic cardiomyopathy: pressure -volume analysis with a nonimaging scintillation probe. Circulation 68:1062–1073, 1983.

25. Bussmann W-D, Hopf R, Trompler A, Kaltenbach M: Hemodynamics and contractility after oral, intravenous and intracoronary application of calcium antagoists. 8:138–147.

26. Hopf R, Kaltenbach M: Einfluss hoher Dosen von Verapamil auf die linksventikuläre Hämody-namik. In: Gross F (ed), Die Bedeutung der Kalzium-Antagonisten für die Hochdrucktherapie. Münchn Med Wschr-Taschenbuch, München, 1984, PP 41–55.

8. Surgical treatment of hypertrophic obstructive cardiomyopathy

H.D. SCHULTE and W. BIRCKS

Abstract. Hypertrophic obstructive cardiomyopaty (HOCM) today can be treated successfully in many cases by using beta adrenergic blocking agents and calcium antagonists. However, a number of patients remain symptomatic and do not respond appropriately to drug therapy. They may become candidates for surgical treatment.

Hemodynamically and morphologically two types of HOCM are to be differentiated: the typical subvalvular and the atypical midventricular or apical myocardial obstruction.

The history of surgical treatment since 1958 describes a variety of approaches and techniques for relief of the left ventricular outflow tract obstruction. Additionally, the actual surgical intervention including myocardial protection is demonstrated in detail.

In a series of 160 surgical patients (1963 to March 31, 1984) 145 patients had typical, 15 atypical HOCM. Our indications for surgery are today:
  1. clinical symptoms according at least clinical class III (NYHA);
  2. no improvement after conservative drug therapy.
Predominantly the transaortic approach and subvalvular and midventricular myectomy were performed. Hospital mortality of the whole surgical series was 7.5% (12 of 160 patients), for typical HOCM 6.9% (10 of 145 patients), for atypical HOCM 13.3% (2 of 15 patients). During the last years (1977 to 1984) operative mortality could be dropped to 5% (6 of 119 patients). The primary intra-operative result of surgical treatment was controlled by determination of the pre- and post-corrective LV and aorta pressure gradients at a normal beat and at a post-extrasystolic beat in 92 patients:

normal beat before: 53 ± 4, after: $9 \pm 1 \,\mathrm{mm\,Hg}$

post-extra-systolic beat before: 118 ± 5, after: $20 \pm 2 \,\mathrm{mm\,Hg}$

The peri-operative complications were divided into those related to the disease and those non-related to the disease and those non-related to HOCM.

Disease related were: severe mitral insufficiency with necessary mitral valve replacement ($n=7$), aortic valve reconstruction ($n=2$), secondary VSD ($n=6$), total av-block ($n=5$), left bundle branch block ($3=37$), cerebral emboli ($n=4$), reoperation of HOCM ($c=3$).

Disease non-related were: intestinal bleeding ($n=2$), pulmonary embolism ($n=2$), rethoracotomy for bleeding complicatons ($n=5$), wound healing problems ($n=2$), post-operative hernia ($n=2$), post-operative endocarditis with double valve replacement ($n=2$) and others.

Although the hospital mortality and peri-operative complication rates are considerable, surgical treatment in symptomatic patients after failing drug therapy is recommended. Long-term post-operative follow-up studies as well as comparative exercise investigations demonstrate in many cases the best clinical results after surgical myectomy.

Introduction

The natural history of patients with hypertrophic obstructive cardiomyopathy (HCOM) clearly indicates a slowly, but steadily progredient clinical course. This statement is based on several clinical long-term observations over years published by Frank [1], Shah [2], Loogen [3, 4], McKenna [5], Kuhn [6] and others. Morphologically and hemodynamically we have to differentiate two types of HOCM which we define as the *typical* subvalvular and the *atypical* midventricular or apical myocardial obstruction.

Special analysis of deaths demonstrates that sudden death mostly occurs in younger people and in strong relation to physical exertion or strain (Krelhaus [7], Maron [8]). After clinical diagnosis and under medical therapy this event seems to occur less often. But usually during later course HOCM patients are terminated by progressing heart failure and less often by sudden death.

Nevertheless, a large number of patients can be managed well for a long time by medical therapy using beta blocking agents (Goodwin [9], Harrison [10]) or calcium antagonists (Kaltenbach [11]). However, a certain number of patients remain who do not respond appropriately to beta blockers and/or calcium antagonist-therapy. For these patients, the possibility of surgical intervention for relief of the subaortic and/or midventricular obstruction of the left ventricle is well established today.

Indication

The indication for surgery grossly depends on clinical and less on hemodynamic criteria. All clinical patients have to belong to class III (NYHA) with no sufficient response to medical therapy (beta blockers and/or calcium antagonists) which usually was performed for several months to evaluate accurately the efficiency of conservative management.

Patients in clinical class IV (NYHA) of HOCM usually have to bear a considerably higher operative risk than patients in class III. The indication for surgery may remain more or less independent from the hemodynamic situation or the pressure gradient between the left ventricle and the aorta, because in most of the patients demonstrating already distinctly increased left ventricular pressures at rest or after extrasystole the progression usually is very slow. Additionally, the risk of sudden death in this group of patients seems to be diminished (Kuhn [12]). These clinical experiences are included in our advice for surgical treatment for the following main reasons:

1. high probability of distinct subjective and hemodynamic long lastig improvement;
2. distinct tendency of reduced late mortality, including sudden death;
3. acceptable operative risk;

4. a relatively low rate of peri-operative complications.

These two last aspects will be discussed later in detail.

An identical indication is advocated for the group of patients with atypical HOCM which in nearly all cases demonstrates an additional subvalvular muscular obstruction. But in these cases the clinical statement is limited because there are only a few patients up to now. For confirmation, more clinical and surgical experience as well as long-term follow-up has to be gained for this special group of patients.

Surgical management

The history of surgical management of HOCM includes a variety of ingeneous approaches and techniques (Table 1).

The first surgical procedure for relief of the left ventricular outflow tract obstruction was performed by Cleland in 1958 in a patient who survived more than twenty years. A long incision was made in the region of the deep bulbospiral muscle, some of which was removed for histological examination. However, there was no really widespread excision of muscle bulk (Bentall [13]).

Morrow and Brockenbrough [14] operated on their first two patients in early 1960, using the technic of Cleland and Bentall. In the first 10 year old patient there was an unsuccessful attempt to resect some of the muscle mass before effective subaortic ventriculomyotomy. In later cases two parallel incisions were made, using a double bladed knife (about 1 cm apart), and after splitting the muscle fibers beneath both incisions the tissue in between was resected [15].

A combined transaortic and trans-left ventricular approach was performed by Kirklin and Ellis [16] for better resection of the subaortic obstructive muscle.

Julian [17, 18] preferred an extensive fish-mouth incision of the left ventricle

Table 1. Surgical management of HOCM

Cleland, Bentall	1958	Transaortic ventriculomyotomy
Morrow, Brockenbrough	1961	Transaortic double ventriculomyotomy, digital splitting, muscle resection
Kirklin, Ellis	1961	Aortic and left ventricular incision, muscle resection
Swan	1963	Aortic and left ventricular incision, cork borer
Julian	1963	Fish mouth type left ventriculotomy
Lillehei, Levy	1963	Trans left atrial approach, anterior mitral leaflet detachment
Dobell, Scott	1964	Trans left atrial approach, anterior mitral leaflet incision
Johnson	1964	Trans left atrial approach, mitral valve replacement
Harken	1964	Transaortic and right ventricular approach
Cooley	1970	Mitral valve replacement without concomitant myotomy or myectomy
Rastan, Koncz, Konno et al.	1975	Aorto-ventriculoplasty
Bernhard, Cooley, Norman	1976	Apico-aortic valved conduit
Shumway	since 1968	Heart transplantation

alone for optimal exposure. This technique has also been used by Senning [19] with excellent clinical results. For resection after transaortic and left ventricular exposure of the obstructive muscle, Swan [20] used a large laboratory cork borer introduced from the apex and finger-guided through the aortotomy.

Dobell and Scott [21] went through the left atrium after left thoracotomy and exposed the subaortic stensosis by incision of the anterior mitral leaflet from its free margin to the mitral valve ring. The same approach was chosen by Lillehei and Levy [22], who detached the anterior mitral leaflet from the annulus, and by Johnson [23] who performed a mitral valve replacement for the first time. Another concept was introduced by Harken [24] who went through a transverse high right ventriculotomy and exposed the subaortic septal bulge to the right ventricle using the transaortic introduced finger and performed the muscular resection from the right ventricle. The same technique was used by Cooley [25].

In 1975 Cooley [26] presented the results of 27 patients with HOCM who had undergone mitral valve replacement without concomitant septal myotomy or myectomy. This procedure should reduce the systolic obstruction caused by the anterior movement of the aortic leaflet of the mitral valve, eliminate the mitral insufficiency, and avoid possible post-operative partial or total left bundle blocks. Many surgeons were not convinced by this argumentation, and Roberts [27] – a cardiac pathologist – headed towards these explanations and considered this technique as unwarranted and dangerous because it neglected the primary cause of the obstruction and, additionally, it introduced the disease of valve replacement with its complications and a higher mortality rate than the basic disease of HOCM. Also Morrow [28] expressed his conviction that the replacement of a normal mitral valve has no role to play in primary treatment of HOCM.

Another possibility for surgical correction of left ventricular outflow tract obstructions by plastic enlargement was introduced by Rastan and Koncz [29] and Konno et al. [30]. This techqniue of aorto-ventriculoplasty may be taken into consideration for necessary HOCM reoperations.

In 1975 Bernhard [31] published a method for relief of congenital obstruction to left ventricular outflow using a ventricular-aorticprosthesis, which (in a very similar technique) was used by Cooley [32] et al. as an apico-abdominal aorta-valved conduit for relief of aortic stenosis.

The last possible method of treatment in patients with severe idiopathic cardiomyopathy under certain circumstances is heart transplantation which was performed with greatest skill, experience, and best results by Shumway et al. [33] since 1968 in more than 250 clinical cases. In the clinical diagnosis of the recipients the group of cardiomyopathies is the second largest group after coronary artery disease.

Actual surgical tecnique

After preparation of cardio-pulmonary bypass including cannulation, intra-operative simultaneous pressure measurements in LA and LV as well as in the aorta and left ventricle are performed during normal and elective post-extrasystolic beats, documenting mitral insufficiency and the gradient between aorta and LV or within the ventricle. After starting ECC a LV vent is established through the upper right pulmonary vein and left atrium. Ay part of myocardial preservation, general perfusion-hypothermia (blood and esophagus temperature 27 °C for at least 5 min) is utilized. After cross clamping the aorta, an oblique incision to the base of the non-coronary sinus is performed, and selective coronary perfusion using crystalloid histidine-tryptophan buffered cardioplegic solution with Kalium-hydrogen-2-oxo-glutarate (Bretschneider [34]) at 4 to 6 °C is administered under pressure and volume control. Details of our method of clinical cardioplegia are presented in Table 2. For optimal visualization of the subaortic myocardial obstruction, the use of a head light for the surgeon is advisable; the operating table is turned downward on the left; additionally, by external counterpressure on the anterior left ventricular wall, the subvalvular septum is nicely exposed. The extent of the obstruction towards the apex can be appreciated with the palpating finger. Special attention is paid to the protection of the usually normal aortic cusps and the mitral valve, including chordae and papillary muscles during the procedure using special retractors and instruments (Fig. 1).

Table 2. Performance of myocardial protection using crystalloid cardioplegic solution (Bretschneider)

General perfusion hypothermia (5 min < 27°C) blood (esophagus) temperature
Cross clamping ascending aorta and oblique incision into the non–coronary sinus

Selected coronary artery perfusion		
with cold HTK-solution (4-6°C):	Na^+	15 mmol/l
and surface cooling of the heart	K^+	10 mmol/l
Coronary perfusion pressure:		
– until cardiac arrest 100 mmHg	Mg^{++}	4 mmol/l
– during cardiac arrest 40 mmHg	CC^-	58 mmol/l
Coronary perfusion time (8 – 10 min)	Histidine	170 mmol/l
Perfusion volume (2000 – 4000 ml)	Histidine–Ce	16 mmol/l
Retrocardial temperature (9 – 15°C)	Tryptophan	2 mmol/l
Calculated myocardial temperature (12 – 15 ° C)	K-hydrogen –	
	2-oxoglutarate	1 mmol/l
Repeated coronary perfusion:		
– after 45 min cross–clamping time; electrical	Mannitol	20 mmol/l
ventricular activity in ECG; high paracoronary	pH (25 °C)	7,2 mmol/l
collateral flow	Osmoliality	290 mosmol/kg

Perfusion pressure reduction of CPB to 40 mmHg for 1 – 2 min. before reopening of the aortic clamp
Postischemic reperfusion time until rewarming (rectal temperature 34 °C) at least 15 – 30 min.

The first myotomy is performed under the apex of the right coronary cusp, perhaps 1 mm to the right but no more, cutting deeply into the obstructing myocardium covered with a distinct layer of fibrotic endocardium in the direction of the apex.

The second myotomy is placed in the same direction, exactly in the commissure between the left and right coronary cusps. The muscle portion between both myotomies is then removed in one piece as far towards the apex as possible creating a deep U-shaped tunnel. Depending on the specific anatomic situation (typical or atypical HOCM extension of the subvalvular obstruction) an additional myotomy can be made into the previous cut channel. Fibrotic and muscular ridges are carefully excised from the rim of the incisions. Special attention is paid to bulging hypertrophic myocardium which might retract the lateral group of chordae during systole, thereby creating mitral insufficiency, and to atypical connections from the papillary muscles and chordae to the muscular septum which are divided. The result of myectomy is controlled by the palpating finger to

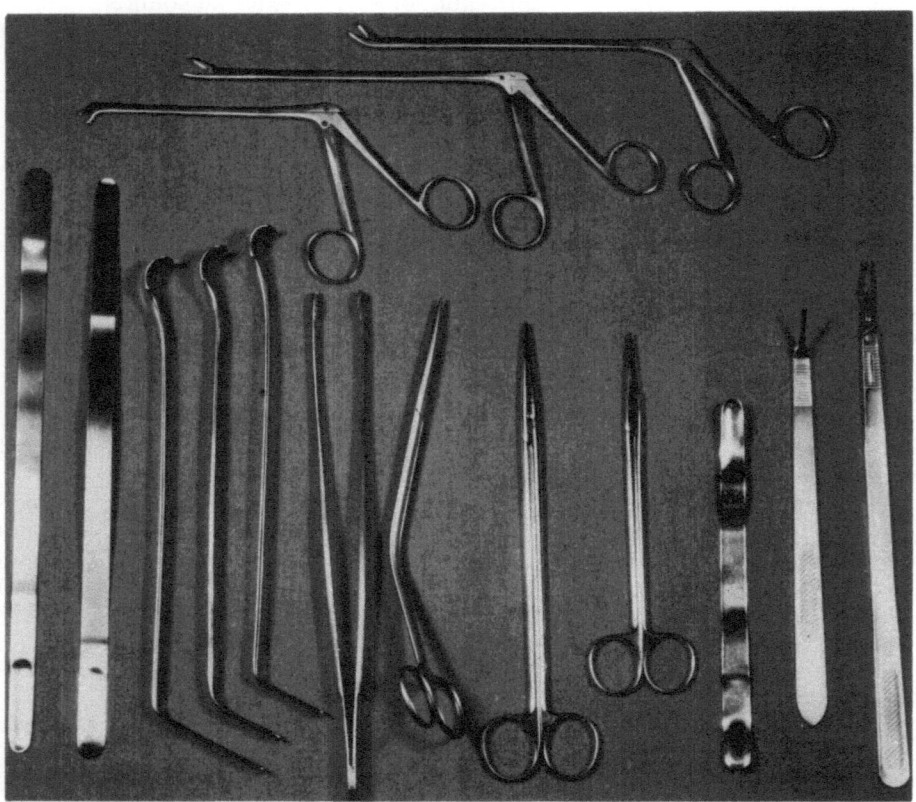

Figure 1.

elucidate residual stenotic myocardium within the created channel for further resection, myotomy, or digital compression and splitting.

In cases of atypical midventricular or apical obstruction, the primary myectomy enables the surgeon to localize and resect deeper obstructions near the base of the papillary muscles. Using longer special angled retractors to expose the septum and to protect the papillary ,muscles, the resection or myotomy can be extended towards the apical region which will further open the ventricular cavity.

In very few special patients with apical obstruction, as for instance in a patient with an additional apical tumor mass, a combined transaortic and trans-left ventricular approach using a fish-mouth type incision may be necessary.

Before closing the aortic incision the ventricular cavity is carefully rinsed with cold Ringer's lactate solution.

After coming off bypass simultaneous measurements of LA and LV, as well as aortic and LV pressures are again performed to ascertain that there is no mitral insufficiency and a sufficient relief of the subvalvular or midventricular obstruction. In case of a considerable residual gradient (aorta-LV) of more than 20 – 30 mmHg or a persistent paradoxical behavior of the aortic and left ventricular pressure a second-look myectomy has to be performed immediately. But before going on bypass again the surgeon has to consider some special factors which may vary the degee of obstruction distinctly, i.e. hypovolemia, position of the pacemaker electrodes in case of intra-operative rhythm disturbances (Table 3).

Patients and findings

From January 10, 1963 to March 31, 1984, a total of 160 patients with HOCM were referred to surgery because of increasing or persistent symptoms despite drug therapy. Except for nine patients in clinical class IV (NYHA), all there surgically treated patients were in clinical class III. The distribution of patients and the hospital deaths (1963 to 1984) are displayed in Table 4, indicating clearly

Table 3. Variability of degree of subvalvular obstruction

Increase:	Hypovolemia, Valsalva maneuver, unfavorable pacemaker lead position, increasing heart rate nitroglycerine rise in myocardial contractility (stress, digitalis, catecholamines)
Decrease:	Anesthesia Hypervolemia beta adrenergic blocking agents, calcium antagonists

Table 4. HOCM – Surgical treatment
(Jan. 10, 1963 to March 31, 1984)

Year	Typical HOCM (n)	Atypical HOCM (n)	Deaths (n)	Total (n)
1963	1	–	–	1
1964	–	–	–	–
1965	3	–	2	3
1966	4	–	1	4
1967	1	–	–	1
1968	–	–	–	–
1969	3	–	–	3
1970	2	–	–	2
1971	4	–	1	4
1972	1	–	–	1
1973	3	–	–	3
1974	5	1	–	6
1975	2	–	1	2
1976	11	–	1	11
1977	10	2	1	12
1978	13	4	–	17
1979	13	3	1	16
1980	12	1	1	13
1981	14	1	–	15
1982	22	2	–	24
1983	17	1	3	18
1984 (March 31)	4	–	–	4
Total	145	15	12 (7.5%)	160

the rising tendency towards surgical treatment since 1976 despite better conservative therapeutic regimens.

The typical and atypical forms of HOCM could be separated pre-operatively by means of cardiological investigation and accurate description of the LV obstructions in the ventriculograms.

According to this differentation the operated patients were assigned to either of these groups (Table 4), resulting in 146 patients with typical and 14 with atypical HOCM. The male: female ratio was nearly 2:1 in both groups.

The mean age of patients was 41 (range 6–72) years in the typical and 48 (range 23–60) years in the atypical category. During the last years the mean age of surgically treated patients has increased distinctly, which suggests that the primary medical treatment could be extended, especially since introduction of the calcium antagonists.

According to the clinical classification (NYHA) 149 patients belonged to class III, and 11 patients were in class IV before surgery. Most of our patients had simple typical (n = 128) or atypical HOCM (n = 10), including a slight degree of mitral insufficiency (class I–II), mostly demonstrated only by systolic regurgitation of contrast medium from the LV into the LA. In 13 patients there was an additional considerable mitral insufficiency which afforded mitral valve replacement in five typical and two atypical cases, which contributed to five perioperative deaths. In one typical HOCM case accidental division of some important chordae tendineæ occurred during myectomy, resulting in massive mitral regurgitation and mitral valve replacement.

Aortic valve disease was present in three patients with typical HOCM. In a 13 year old boy a commissurotomy was possible and effective. A 22 year old woman had a class III aortic insufficiency and a rudimentary subvalvular fibrotic membrane above the typical muscular obstruction. A 37 year old man demonstrated HOCM and severe aortic insufficiency after endocarditis resulting in aortic valve replacement. Another 37 year old patient with typical HOCM late post–operatively developed bacterial endocarditis with severe aortic and mitral insufficiency requiring emergency double valve replacement at another university hospital (Table 5).

Additional symptomatic coronary artery disease was found in 6 patients who underwent aorto-coronary bypass procedures and a resection of a ventricular aneurysm. In this case the subvalvular muscular resection was performed via the anterior-apical ventricular incision.

An unique situation was found in a 39 year old patient with subvalvular and predominant midventricular obstruction as well as a tumor mass filling the apical area of the left ventricle. Surgical correction was performed by transaortic and trans-left ventricular myectomy and removal of the well organized, wall–adherent tumor which histologically proved to be an old thrombus.

Table 5. Typical subaortic and atypical midventricular HOCM
(Jan. 10, 1963 to March 31, 1984)

	Typical HOCM	Atypical HOCM
Patients (n)	145	15
Male: Female	96:49	10:5
Mean age (range) (years)	41 (6–72)	48 (23–60)
Clinical classification III	135	14
(NYHA) IV	10	1
HOCM	128	10
HOCM + mitral valve disease	10 (3+)	3 (2+)
HOCM + aortic valve disease	3	0
HOCM + coronary artery disease	4 RCA	2 RCA
	RCA	RCA + LAD
	RCA + R.marg.	
	RCA+LAD+R.marg. I,II,III	
HOCM + apical thrombus		1
Hospital mortality	10 (6.9%)	2 (13.3%)

Table 6. Distribution of primary operative procedures and related peri–operative mortality.

Procedures	Total		Typical HOCM		Atypical HOCM	
	(n)	(%)	(n)	(%)	(n)	(%)
Transaortic myectomy	130	5 (3.8%)	122	5	8	–
Transaortic + transventricular (LV)	3	1	1	1	2	–
Transaortic + transventricular (RV)	4	1	4	1	–	–
Transaortic + LV + RV (VSD)	1	–	–	–	1	–
Transaortic + MVR	7	5	5	3	2	2
Transaortic + mitral valve reconstruction	2	–	2	–	–	–
Transaortic + AVR	2	–	2	–	–	–
Transaortic + aortic valve reconstruction	3	–	3	–	–	–
Transaortic + CABG	6	–	4	–	2	–
Transventricular (LV) myectomy	2	–	2	–	–	–
Total	160	12 (7.5%)	145	10 (6.9%)	15	2 (13.3%)

The distribution of primary operative procedures for typical and atypical HOCM including the peri–operative mortality are summarized in a table (Table 6). The most performed and favored procedure is the transaortic myectomy which also indicates the lowest mortality rate (3.8%).

Two patients operated in 1965 died because of LV failure; one patient operated in 1980 died after fatal pulmonary embolism on the 13th post–operative day, a complication we did not see before in a paient after ECC. The heart weight at autopsy was nearly 1000 g. A 50 year old woman died suddenly on the 10th p.o. day in 1983 after an exciting telephone call with her family.

The last patient, a 62 year old woman, died after a post–operative rupture of the ascending aorta and massive bleeding in the ICU on the day of surgery (1983).

This analysis of deaths after transaortic myectomy alone indicates that only two earlier patients died and one patient with sudden death in strong relation to the original disease (LV failure, sudden death). A disastrous outcome with only two survivors was found in our seven patients requiring mitral valve replacement.

A 45 year old woman was operated 1975 in cardiogenic shock as an ultima ratio indication; she died intra–operatively after transaortic myectomy, MVR because of increasing mitral insufficiency, and intra–operative support perfusion for nearly 4 h.

A 57 year old woman with atypical HOCM and coronary artery sclerosis, mild mitral insufficiency developed after transaortic myectomy, an increasing mitral insufficiency which could not be treated with a Wooler–plasty. After MVR and LV failure, massive bleeding occurred after heart massage, and she died intra–operatively.

A 52 year old woman showed signs of LV failure 7 days after transaortic myectomy and after a bradycardia a circulatory arrest occurred. As she could not be resuscitated, she was taken to the operating theatre and put on bypass again as an emergency procedure. Pressure tracings after a considerable time of reperfusion demonstrated massive mitral and tricuspid regurgitation and MVR was performed. Shortly after a rethoracotomy because of bleeding problems she died on the day of surgery in LV failure.

Two additional patients died on the 10th and 48th post–operative day because of LV failure and several post–operative complications such as respiratory insufficiency, gastro–intestinal bleeding, arrhythmias, and perivalvular leakage.

The poor results with MVR do not have to be considered as unavoidable. Perhaps we have not been aggressive enough to replace the mitral valve in cases with additional acquired mitral lesions.

Nevertheless, the hospital mortality in our surgical series decreased distinctly with growing experience over four time-periods (Table 7). All patients were operated by two surgeons or one of them as first assistant in 11 patients.

Table 7. Hospital mortality for HOCM–surgical series

Periods of experience	Patients (n)	Mortality (n) (%)
1963 – 1969	12	3 (25,0%)
1970 – 1976	29	3 (10,3%)
1977 – 1980	58	3 (5,2%)
1981 – 1984 (March 31)	61	3 (4,9%)
Total	160	12 (7,5%)

Intra–operative hemodynamic results

In all patients the systolic pressure gradient between left ventricle and aorta during normal beats and after a post–extrasystolic beat is measured and documented before and after myectomy. The systolic pressure gradients and the paradoxical post–extrasystolic behavior of the LV and aortic pressures (Brockenbrough phenomenon) could be abolished or at least considerably reduced. In 15 patients the control after myectomy indicated a high residual gradient (30 mm Hg) which caused immediately a second look procedure with additional resection of subvalvular obstructive myocardium which usually led to a much better hemodynamic result.

In a group of patients (n = 92) with accurate pressure tracings before and after myectomy, the final intra–operative result is documented during a normal heart beat and a post–extrasystolic beat (Table 8).

Table 8. Intra–operative pressure gradients before and after myectomy
(n = 92)

	Gradient before myectomy	Gradient after
	Mean ± SD (mm Hg)	Mean ± SD (mm Hg)
Normal beat	53 ± 4	9 ± 1
Post–extrasystolic beat	118 ± 5	20 ± 2

Peri–operative complications

Peri–operative complications can be considered as related to the disease or to the special procedure, or non-related (Table 9).

Two minor procedure–related aortic valve injuries of the cusps could be reconstructed with good long–term results. The subvalvular resection caused a septal communication to the right ventricle in six patients. In one patient the VSD was detected and closed via right ventriculotomy during the primary intervention. Another patient had reoperation 6 weeks later for closure of the defect. In the other four patients the VSD is very small and no surgical repair is needed.

Three patients had to be reoperated because of continuing outflow tract obstruction. The reason is not a recidive, but an insufficient relief of the subvalvular obstruction at the primary intervention. This concerns our first operated patient out of 1963, who was reoperated in 1971 and died on the 9th post–operative day because of LV failure. Both other patients could be reoperated successfully in 1978 and 1983 without any additional problems.

In six patients a procedure–related total AV-block resulted, which was treated for the first 10 to 16 days by using the transthoracic epimyocardial pacemaker leads. Two patients died on the 8th and 9th post–operative day, and in four patients a permanent pacemaker system was implanted.

The incidence of post–operative left bundle branch block (LBBB) increased continously during the last years, which coincides with our surgical efforts to improve the efficacy of the procedure, by means of more extended myocardial resection. According to Maron [35] and our limited experience, LBBB seems to have no negative influence on the immediate surgical outcome and the long–term results.

The main complications not related to HOCM and their outcomes are summarized in part B of Table 9, giving a general spectrum of common hazards for thoracic and cardiac surgery. But it should be mentioned that septicemia, gastrointestinal bleeding, and hepatitis B belong to the first two periods of surgical experience (1963 – 1976).

Table 9. Peri–operative complications

A. Related to HOCM or special surgical procedure	
Mitral valve replacement	7 (5+)
Aortic valve injury (reconstructed)	2
Secondary VSD	6
Reoperation for HOCM	3 (1+)
Ventricular wall perforation	1 (+)
Septal infarction	1
Total av-block (pacemaker–implantation)	5
Left bundle branch block	37
Right bundle branch block	1
Cerebral emboli	4
B. Non–related to HOCM or special surgical procedure	
Rupture of ascending aorta	1 (+)
Septicemia	1 (+)
Intestinal bleeding	2 (1+)
Pulmonary embolism	2 (1+)
Rethoracotomy (bleeding)	5
Wound healing problems	2
Post–operative hernia	2
Pericardial effusion	1
Acute renal failure	2
Hepatitis B	3

Discussion

After more than 25 years of surgical treatment of HOCM, the question of whether medical or surgical treatment in a particular patient should be preferred is not yet decided definitely. But the general rule that each patient with symptomatic HOCM should be treated first conservatively is widely accepted. Only in case of inadequate response to differentiated drug therapy must surgery be taken into consideration, using the well–established technique of ventricular septal myotomy and myectomy.

A synopsis of some early operative results since 1974 demonstrates clearly a very similar experience in some surgical centers interested in HOCM and published during the last ten years (Table 10). Nevertheless, the early mortality rate has to be reduced; this can be achieved by further experience. But we have to realize that surgical treatment in nearly all clinical cases seems to be one good chance after the failing of medical therapy in severely symptomatic patients. And therefore reports on the long–term efficacy of early successful surgical interventions are of utmost importance.

The largest and excellent documented series of the Bethesda group was reported by Maron [35], reviewing 240 out of 280 patients operated before 1980. After

Table 10. Early operative results (hospital mortality)

Author	Year	Patients (n)	Mortality (%)
Bigelow [36]	1974	39	7.5
Tajik [37]	1974	43	16
Björk [38]	1976	32	6.3
Cooley [25]	1976	27	3.7
Senning [19]	1976	39	2.6
Agnew [39]	1977	49	4.1
Maron [35]	1983	240	8
Binet [40]	1983	76	9.2
Rothlin [41]	1983	64	1.6
Düsseldorf	1963–1984 (March 31)	160	7.5
	1977–1984	119	5

consequent post–operative follow–up, 70% of the patients had improved symptomatically; only 9% had persistent or recurrent considerable functional limitation, whereas 7% died during the 19 year follow–up because of the original disease. Another large experience of 254 patients was evaluated by Goodwin and Oakley [42].

Binet [40], in his series of 76 out of 123 patients operated between 1964 and 1982, found an annual death rate of 3.7% which seems to be acceptable in relation to a patient group selected by the severity of their illness and the failure of prior medical therapy. Clinical prognostic studies of Kuhn [6] confirmed that the cumulative survival rates are significantly higher in surgical patients with typical HOCM than in those treated conservatively.

A clinical consecutive comparison of 15 years of surgical versus medical treatment was performed by Rothlin [41] which resulted, for instance, in a 10 year mortality rate of 80% in the surgical and 71% in the non–surgical series. The most common cause of death in the non–surgical series was sudden death, in the surgical group congestive heart failure, which late post–operatively was related to myocardial injury as a late consequence of septal myectomy.

Losse [43] performed some exercise investigations in patients with HOCM to evaluate the clinical and hemodynamic effects of medical therapy with propranolol and verapamil, and surgical treatment (transaortic subvalvular myectomy). These exercise measurements demonstrated calcium antagonist therapy to be more effective than propranolol administration. But the best results concerning clinical symptoms, exercise capacity, and exercise hemodynamics where achieved after surgical myectomy.

To date these few reports on long–term evaluations after medical and surgical therapy seem to indicate that our policy of HOCM treatment and operative indication since many years can be confirmed by the experience of some other distinguished investigators. These results gathered and gained over nearly 25 years in several centers indicate preference for medical therapy in patients with HOCM, using preferably the calcium antagonist verapamil. However, in non-responding and symptomatic patients in clinical class III NYHA, a surgical intervention with acceptable early results and a fair clinical long-term prognosis is the therapy of choice today.

References

1. Frank MJ, Abdulla FAM, Canedo MI, Saylors RE: Long-term management of hypertrophic obstructive cardiomyopathy. Am J Cardiol 42: 993, 1978.
2. Shah PM, Adelman AG, Wigle ED, Gobel FL, Bruchell HB: The natural (and unnatural) history of hypertrophic obstructive cardiomyopathy. Circ Res 34/35 Suppl 2: 179, 1974.
3. Loogen G, Kuhn H, Krelhaus W: Natural history of hypertrophic cardiomyopathy and the effects of therapy. In: Kaltenbach M, Loogen F, Olsen EGJ (eds), Cardiomyopathy and myocardial biopsy. Springer Berlin, 1978, pp 286–299.
4. McKenna WJ, Deanfield J, Faruqui A, England D, Oakley C, Goodwin JF: Prognosis in hypertrophic cardiomyopathy: role of age and clinical, electrocardiographic and hemodynamic features. Am J Cardiol 47: 432, 1981.
5. Loogen F, Kuhn H, Gietzen B, Lo\u0161se B, Schulte HD, Bircks W: Clinical course and prognosis of patients with typical and atypical hypertrophic obstructive and with hypertrophic non–obstructive cardiomyopathy. Eur Heart J 4 (suppl) 145 – 153, 1983.
6. Kuhn H, Gietzen F, Mercier J, Lo\u0161se B, Ko\u0148ler E, Schulte HD, Bircks W, Loogen F: Studies of the clinical picture, course, and prognosis of different forms of hypertrophic cardiomyopathy. Z Kardiol 72: 83 – 98, 1983.
7. Krelhaus W, Kuhn H, Loogen F: Analysis of deaths in the course of hypertrophic obstructive cardiomyopathy. In: Kaltenbach M, Loogen F, Olsen EGJ (eds), Cardiomyopathy and myocardial biopsy. Springer, Berlin 1978, pp 300 – 307.
8. Maron BJ, Epstein SE, Roberts WC: Hypertrophic cardiomyopathy: a common cause of sudden death in the young competitive athlete. Eur Heart J 4 (suppl): 135 – 144, 1983.
9. Goodwin JF, Shah PM, Oakley CM, Cohen J, Yipintsoi T, Pocock W: Clinical pharmacology of hypertrophic obstructive cardiomyopathy. In: Wolstenholm GEW, O'Connor M (eds), CIBA foundation symposium on cardiomyopathies. Little, Brown & Co, Boston, 1964, p 189.
10. Harrison DC, Braunwald E, Glick G, Mason DT, Chidsey CA, Ross Jr J: Effects of beta adrenergic blockade on circulation with particular reference to observations in patients with hypertrophic subaortic stenosis. Circulation 29: 84, 1964.
11. Kaltenbach M, Hopf R, Keller M: Calciumantagonistische Therapie bei hypertroph- obstruktiver Kardiomyopathie. Dtsch Med Wschr 101: 1284, 1976.
12. Kuhn H, Krelhaus W, Bircks W, Schulte HD, Loogen F: Indication for surgical treatment in patients with hypertrophic obstructive cardiomyopathy. In: Kaltenbach M, Loogen F, Olsen EGJ (eds), Cardiomyopathy and myocardial biopsy. Springer, Berlin–Heidelberg–New York, 1978, pp 308 – 315.
13. Bentall HH: The place of surgery in hypertrophic obstructive cardiomyopathy (idiopathic hypertrophic subaortic stenosis). J Thorac Cardiovasc Surg 51: 49 – 52, 1966.
14. Morrow AG, Brockenbrough: Surgical treatment of idiopathic hypertrophic subaortic stenosis: technic and hemodynamic results of subaortic ventriculomyotomy. Ann Surg 154: 181 – 189, 1961.
15. Morrow AG, Lambrew CT, Braunwald E: Idiopathic hypertrophic subaortic stenosis II. Opera-

tive treatment and the results of pre- and post–operative hemodynamic evaluations. Circulation 29/30 (suppl IV): 120 – 151, 1964.

16. Kirklin JW, Ellis FW: Surgical relief of diffuse subvalvular aortic stenosis. Circulation 24: 739, 1961.

17. Julian OC, Quoted by Morrow [14].

18. Julian OC, Dye WS, Javid H, Hunter JA, Muenster JJ, Najati H: Apical left ventriculotomy in subaortic stenosis due to a fibromuscular hypertrophy. Circulation 31/32 (suppl I): 45, 1965.

19. Senning A: Transventricular relief of idiopathic hypertrophic subaortic stenosis. J Cardiovasc Surg 17: 371 – 375, 1976.

20. Swan H: Subaortic muscular stenosis: a new surgical technique for repair. J Thorac, Cardiovasc Surg 47: 681, 1964.

21. Dobell ARC, Scott AJ: Hypertrophic subaortic stenosis. Evolution of a surgical technique. J Thorac Cardiovas Surg 47: 26, 1964.

22. Lillehei CW, Levy MJ: Transatrial exposure for correction of subaortic stenosis. JAMA 186: 8, 1963.

23. Johnson J: (1964): In discussion of Dobell and Scott [21].

24. Harken DE (1964): In discussion of Dobell and Scott [21].

25. Cooley DA, Beall Jr AC, Hallman GL: Obstructive lesions of the left ventricular outflow tract: surgical treatment. Circulation 31: 612, 1965.

26. Cooley DA, Wukasch DC, Leachman RD: Mitral valve replacement for idiopathic subaortic stenosis. Results in 27 patients. J Cardiovasc Surg 17: 380 – 387, 1976.

27. Roberts WC: Operative treatment of hypertrophic obstructive cardiomyopathy. The case against mitral valve replacement. Am J Cardiol 32: 377, 1973.

28. Morrow AG: Hypertrophic aortic stenosis. Operative methods utilized to relieve left ventricular outflow obstruction. J Thorac Cardiovasc Surg 76: 423 – 430, 1978.

29. Rastan H, Koncz J: Plastische Erweiterung des linken Ausflußtraktes – eine neue Operationsmethode. Thoraxchir 3: 169 – 175, 1975.

30. Konno S, Imai Y, Jida Y, Makajima M, Tetsuno K: A new method for prosthetic valve replacement in congenital aortic stenosis associated with hypoplasia of the aortic ring. J Thorac Cardiovasc Surg 70: 109, 1975.

31. Bernhard FW, Poirier V, La Farge CG: Relief of congenital obstruction to left ventricular outflow with a ventricular–aortic prosthesis. J Thorac Cardiovasc Surg 69: 223, 1975.

32. Cooley DA, Norman JC, Mullins CE, Grace RR: Left ventricle to abdominal aorta conduits for relief of aortic stenosis. Cardiovasc Dis 2: 376, 1975.

33. Stinson EB, Shumway NE: Transplantation of the heart. In: Longmore DB (ed), Modern Cardiac Surgery. MTP-Press Limited, Lancaster, 1978, pp 3–18.

34. Bretschneider HJ: Myocardial protection. J Thorac Cardiovasc Surg 28: 295, 1980.

35. Maron BJ, Epstein SE, Morrow AG: Symptomatic status and prognosis of patients after operation for hypertrophic obstructive cardiomyopathy: efficacy of ventricular septal myotomy and myectomy. Eur Heart J 4 (suppl F): 175 – 185, 1983.

36. Bigelow WG, Trimble AS, Wigle DE, Adelman AG, Felderhof SE: The treatment of muscular subaortic stenosis. J Thorac Cardiovasc Surg 68: 384 – 390, 1974.

37. Tajik AJ, Giuliani ER, Weidmann WH, Brandenburg RO, McGoon DC: Idiopathic hypertrophic subaortic stenosis, long–term surgical follow–up. Am J Cardiol 34: 815, 1974.

38. Bjork VD, Radegran K: Obstructive cardiomyopathy. J Cardiovasc Surg 17: 376 – 379, 1976.

39. Agnew TM, Barrat–Boyes GB, Brandt PT, Roibe AHG, Loewe JB, O'Brian KP: Surgical resection in idiopathic hypertrophic subaortic stenosis with a combined approach through aorta and left ventricle. A long–term follow–up study in 49 patients. J Thorac Cardiovasc Surg 74: 307 – 316, 1977.

40. Binet JP, David P, Piot JD: Surgical treatment of hypertrophic obstructive cardiomyopathies. Eur Heart J 4 (suppl F): 191 – 195, 1983.

41. Rothlin ME, Gobet D, Haberer T, Krayenbuehl HP, Turina M, Senning A: Surgical treatment versus medical treatment in hypertrophic obstructive cardiomyopathy. Eur Heart J 4 (suppl F): 215 – 223, 1983.
42. Goodwin JF, Oakley CM: Medical and surgical treatment of hypertrophic cardiomyopathy. Eur Heart J 4 (suppl F): 209 – 215, 1983.
43. Loŝse B, Kuhn H, Loogen F, Schulte HD: Exercise performance in hypertrophic cardiomyopathies. Eur Heart J 4 (suppl F): 197 – 208, 1983.

9. Pathophysiologic mechanisms responsible for the clinical spectrum of hypertrophic cardiomyopathy

S.E. EPSTEIN, B.J. MARON, R.O. BONOW, D.R. ROSING
and R.O. CANNON, III

The pathophysiologic mechanisms contributing to the hemodynamic and clinical manifestations of hypertrophic cardiomyopathy (HCM) involve abnormalities affecting both systolic and diastolic function, as well as myocardial perfusion. In addition, not only is the interaction of these abnormalities complex, but the degree to which each contributes to the clinical presentations of individual patients may differ markedly. These factors have led to many misconceptions concerning the pathophysiologic mechanisms causally related to the production of symptoms in HCM, and therefore how best to treat this disease. In this manuscript we will review some of the studies we have performed in the Cardiology Branch of the National Heart, Lung, and Blood Institute over the past several years that help contribute to our understanding of this fascinating disease.

Patterns of hypertrophy and relation to clinical and hemodynamic findings

One of the characteristic morphologic abnormalities of HCM is a ventricular septum that is hypertrophied out of proportion to the free left ventricular wall [104]. Although asymetric septal hypertrophy (ASH) was initially believed to be one of the essential markers of HCM, subsequent 2–dimensional echocardiography has demonstrated the enormous diversity of the patterns of hypertrophy present in this disease [5, 6]. Figure 1 shows some of these patterns, as detected by cross–sectional 2–D images of the left ventricle.

While the large majority of HCM patients do have hypertrophy of the anterior septum, myocardial thickening often involves other portions of the left ventricle to a great or greater degree as found in the anterior septum. Occasionally there can be true concentric hypertrophy, and in some patients hypertrophy only involves areas of the heart other than the anterior septum (Type IV, Fig. 1). This latter situation is of diagnostic importance, since, if hypertrophy involves portions of the heart inaccessible to the M–mode echo beam (the posterior septum,

134

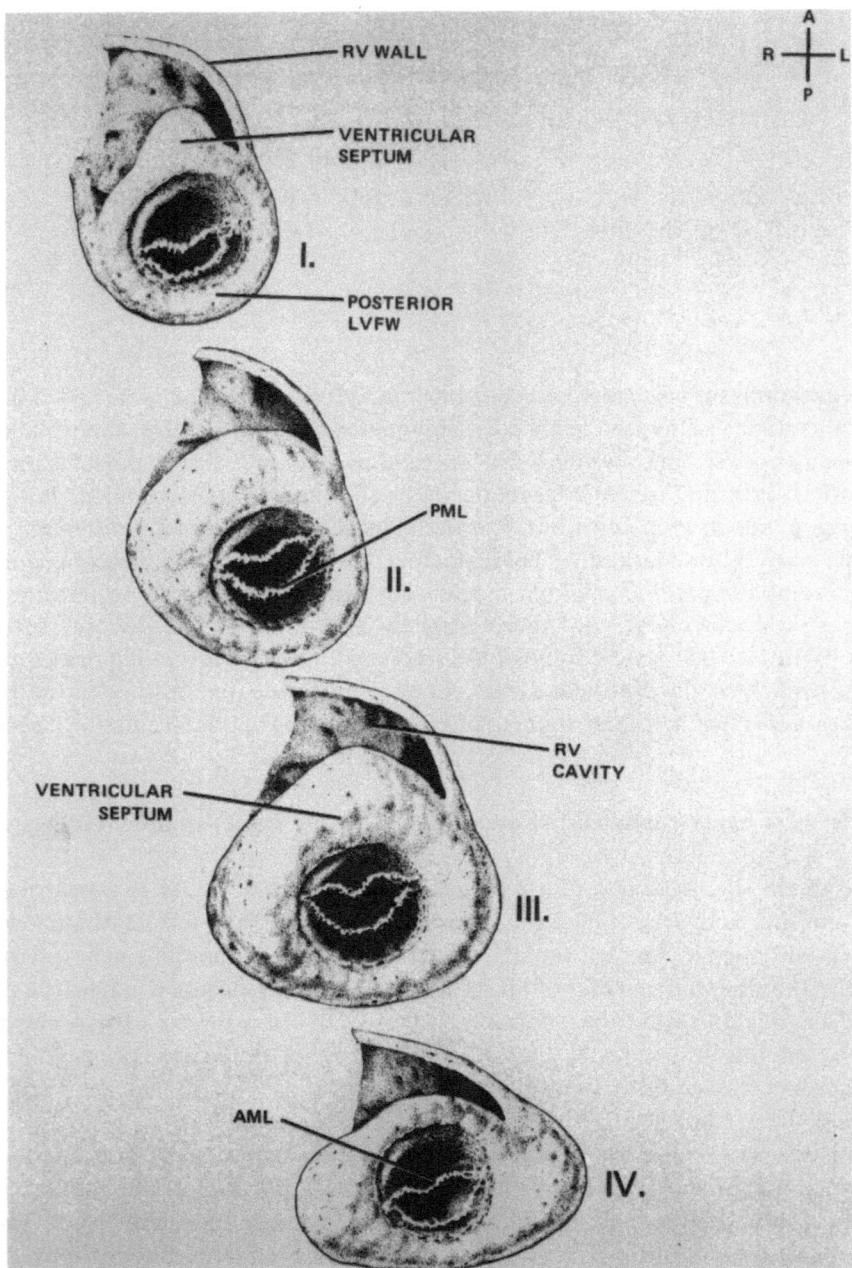

Figure 1. Artistic representation of four patterns of left ventricular hypertrophy identified with wide angle two dimensional echocardiography in patients with hypertrophic cardiomyopathy. Shown only are cross–sectional planes at the level of the mitral valve. AML = anterior mitral leaflet; LVFW = left ventricular free wall; PML = posterior mitral leaflet; RV = right ventricular; other abbreviations as before.

cardiac apex, or anterolateral left ventricular wall), M–mode echocardiography may be entirely normal.

The different patterns of hypertrophy are of some pathophysiologic importance. For example, although it is not known whether they relate to prognosis, patients with the more extensive patterns of hypertrophy (i.e., involving the entire septum and lateral wall of the left ventricle) have a greater likelihood of having severe symptoms than patients in whom the hypertrophy is more limited [6]. Similarly, the distribution of hypertrophy influences the likelihood that outflow obstruction exists. When the anterior septum is hypertrophied, significant (≥ 30 mm Hg) gradients are detected across the left ventricular outflow tract much more commonly than when hypertrophy is limited to portions of the left ventricle other than the anterior septum [6]. This finding is consistent with the pathophysiologic mechanisms believed to cause left ventricular outflow obstruction [7, 8]. The extensive hypertrophy of the anterior septum contributes to narrowing of the left ventricular outflow tract, which is bordered by the ventricular septum and anterior leaflet of the mitral valve. The narrowed outflow tract causes the velocity of blood flow in this region to increase, predisposing to the development of Venturi forces and thereby to the anterior motion of the mitral valve during systole (SAM). The interposition of the mitral valve into the left ventricular outflow tract presents the contracting left ventricle with a mechanical impediment to emptying.

Pathophysiologic mechanisms contributing to abnormalities in left ventricular function

There are probably at least three major mechanisms contributing to abnormal left ventricular function and to symptoms in patients with HCM: (1). abnormal diastolic function, (2) myocardial ischemia and (3). obstruction to left ventricular outflow.

Critical to an understanding of the pathophysiology of this disease is the concept that the relative contribution of each of those mechanisms to symptoms may vary markedly from one patient to another, and that the optimal therapeutic approach to a given patient will depend on which one or combination of these mechanisms is the major factor responsible for precipitating the patient's symptoms.

Abnormal diastolic function

Most patients with HCM have one or more manifestations of abnormal diastolic dysfunction, which result from abnormalities in either left ventricular distensibility, left ventricular relaxation, or both [9]. Left ventricular distensibility is determined by the relation between left ventricular pressure and volume changes occurring during the diastolic phase of the cardiac cycle. An increase in myocardial mass can increase stiffness (decrease distensibility) of the left ventricle [10, 11], which will lead to a steeper slope of the left ventricular pressure–volume relation, so that left ventricular diastolic pressure is higher for any degree of left ventricular filling, as compared to the relation exhibited by an individual with a normal left ventricle. Left ventricular relaxation is also abnormally long in patients with HCM, as manifest by a prolonged isovolumic relaxation period and a reduced rate at which left ventricular pressure declines [12–14].

There is a complex relationship between left ventricular distensibility and left ventricular relaxation. For example, prolonged relaxation results in increased myocardial tension extending into the phase of early diastolic filling. The increased tension shifts the left ventricular diastolic pressure–volume relation, so that left ventricular distensibility is reduced. The net result of these abnormalities is to impair left ventricular filling [13–16] and raise left ventricular diastolic pressure for any diastolic volume.

Abnormal left ventricular diastolic function predisposes to reduced cardiac output and elevated left ventricular filling pressures, and thereby undoubtedly contributes to the development of symptoms in patients with HCM. It also appears that the salutary symptomatic effects produced by some therapeutic interventions are due, at least in part, to their capacity to improve diastolic function. For example, Fig. 2 depicts the results of a short course of oral verapamil on the filling characteristics of a patient with HCM, as determined by radionuclide angiography. Compared to normals, peak filling rate is markedly diminished and the interval from end–systole to peak filling rate is prolonged. During verapamil therapy, a marked improvement in both of these filling parameters can be appreciated both at rest and during exercise. We have observed these salutary effects on early diastolic filling in the majority of patients with HCM treated with verapamil [15, 16]. We have also noted a correlation between verapamil–induced improvement in diastolic function and verapamil–induced improvement in exercise capacity, both short term (1 week – 1 month) and long term (1–2 years). Thus, during long term studies 91% of patients in whom verapamil persistently improved peak filling rate, demonstrated a persistent increase in treadmill exercise capacity related to pre–verapamil values, whereas only 14% of patients not demonstrating an improved peak filling rate following verapamil exhibited enhanced exercise capacity while on the drug [17]. These data provide strong evidence that abnormalities in diastolic filling can contribute importantly to symptoms in patients with HCM and that one of the mechanisms by which verapamil improves symptoms is by improving diastolic function.

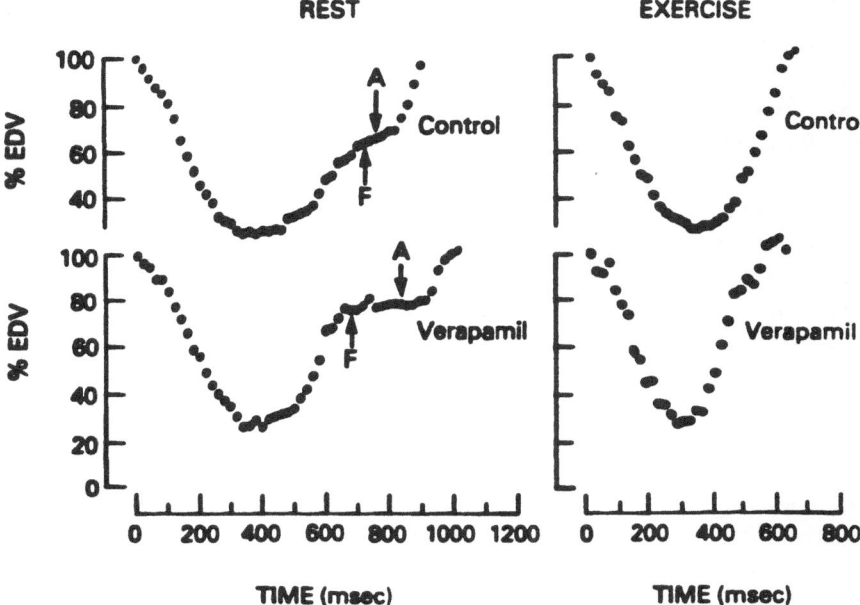

Figure 2. Left ventricular volume curves by radionuclide angiography at rest and during exercise in a patient with hypertrophic cardiomyopathy. Oral verapamil (480 mg/day) results in enhanced diastolic filling at rest: a shortened isvolumic relaxation phase, an increased rate and extent of rapid diastolic filling, and a reduced contribution of atrial systole to total filling volume. Increased rate of filling is also evident during exercise. Each point represents 20 msec (reproduced with permission from Am J Cardiol).

Myocardial ischemia

There are several ways by which myocardial ischemia can occur in patients with HCM. Occasionally, patients with HCM and angina pectoris have coexisting coronary artery disease. However, angina is a common symptom in this disease even in younger patients and in such cases is not usually associated with underlying atherosclerotic heart disease. Moreover, extensive myocardial scarring is not uncommonly observed in patients dying with hypertrophic cardiomyopathy; the scar is actually transmural in about 15% of autopsied patients [18]. Patients with extensive scarring did not have associated extramural coronary occlusive disease, and the areas of myocardial necrosis were not selectively limited to the areas of distribution of the extramural coronary arteries.

In the absence of epicardial coronary artery disease, ischemia may develop in HCM as a result of several other possible mechanisms. First, a substantial number of patients with HCM who die, have been found to have structural abnormalities of the intramyocardial coronary arteries, including medial hypertrophy and intimal hyperplasia, leading to an apparent reduction in the lumen of these vessels [19]. It is quite likely that such lesions diminish the maximal vasodilator capacity and thereby compromise the ability of the coronary circulation to augment flow appropriately in response to increased myocardial metabolic demands.

Second, there is evidence in experimental models of left ventricular hypertrophy that hypertrophy can outstrip the capacity of capillaries to supply oxygen. Thus, myocardial hypertrophy reduces maximal vasodilator capacity [20], and capillary density per unit myocardial mass in hypertrophied myocardium is reduced when compared to that observed in normal hearts [21], suggesting that capillaries do not proliferate enough to keep pace with the proliferation of myocardial tissue. The resulting increase in intercapillary distances might lead to inadequate diffusion of oxygen to those portions of myocardium furthest from a capillary, causing ischemia and angina.

Third, it is likely that the elevated filling pressures found so commonly in HCM may contribute to the precipitation or exacerbation of myocardial ischemia. Thus, it has been shown experimentally that there is an indirect correlation between left ventricular filling pressure and maximal coronary flow; under experimental conditions in which maximal coronary flow is achieved by infusion of adenosine, as left ventricular filling pressure increases, coronary flow decreases [22]. It has also been shown in patients with HCM that when heart rate is increased by pacing to levels that cause elevated filling pressures, myocardial blood flow decreases [23]. Elevated filling pressures presumably translate into increased compressive forces on the coronary vasculature, thereby decreasing the cross–sectional area of the intramyocardial vessels and increasing coronary vascular resistance.

Left ventricular outflow tract obstruction

Questions have been raised as to whether true obstruction to left ventricular outflow in patients with HCM exists. Investigators doubting the presence of obstruction despite the measurement of a large gradient [24–29] argue that an impedance to left ventricular outflow cannot be present in a ventricle that empties rapidly and in which there is often virtual obliteration of the apical portions of the cavity by end–systole.

However, there are several observations that appear to us to point almost incontrovertably to the conclusion that the presence of a gradient in a patient with HCM usually is an indication of true obstruction to left ventricular outflow [29–42]. First, the anterior leaflet of the mitral valve moves forward into the left ventricular outflow tract during the first third of systole; hence, a potential mechanical impediment to left ventricular outflow exists. That this actually does mechanically interfere with ejection is strongly suggested by the fact that the onset of contact between the mitral valve and ventricular septum coincides very closely with (1) a rapid deceleration of blood flow velocity as measured in the ascending aorta, (2) premature partial closure of the aortic valve leaflets, and (3) the development of a subaortic intraventricular pressure gradient.

Additional evidence favoring the concept of outflow obstruction [42] is that (1) left ventricular ejection patterns of patients with obstructive HCM differ markedly from the patterns recorded from patients without obstruction and from normal individuals, (2) the left ventricle continues to contract and shorten after the onset of mitral–septal apposition and the development of the gradient and, (3) on average, nearly half of the volume of blood that is ultimately ejected from the left ventricle is ejected *after* the onset of mitral–septal apposition and development of the outflow tract gradient. Finally, the clinical importance of left ventricular outflow obstruction is strongly indicated by the fact that in patients with HCM and obstruction, left ventricular myotomy–myectomy usually leads to marked symptomatic improvement [43–48]. In this operation, about two grams of tissue from the basal ventricular septum are removed which, by substantially increasing the very small cross–sectional area of the left ventricular outflow tract of patients with obstructive HCM [49], reduces or eliminates the gradient. While the fall in outflow gradient occurs in virtually all patients operated upon, left ventricular filling pressures do not decrease consistently [43, 44]. Although alternative mechanisms can be posed to explain the improved exercise capacity and symptoms exhibited by most patients following surgery, the simplest one, which is at the same time entirely consistent with the hemodynamic data, is that salutary effects occur because the marked reduction in left ventricular outflow obstruction leads to marked decreases in left ventricular systolic pressures.

Potential mechanisms responsible for specific symptoms in HCM patients

On the basis of the preceding discussion, it would appear that the pathophysiologic causes of the symptoms present in patients with HCM are multiple. The most common symptoms experienced by patients with this disease (excluding those due to arrhythmias) are angina pectoris, exertional dyspnea, and syncope or near–syncope. Each of the pathophysiologic mechanisms proposed – abnormal diastolic function, myocardial ischema, and obstruction to LV outflow –can lead, through different pathophysiologic pathways, to the same symptom complexes. Thus, impaired diastolic function (1) can cause pulmonary congestion and thereby dyspnea by increasing left ventricular filling pressure, (2) can cause angina by increasing intramyocardial compressive forces and thereby interfere with coronary flow, and (3) can cause syncope or near–syncope by interfering with cardiac filling and thereby predisposing to reduced cardiac output with resultant hypotension. Likewise, ischemia (1) can cause pulmonary congestion and dyspnea by impairing diastolic or systolic function, and thereby increase left ventricular filling pressures, (2) can result in angina and (3) cause syncope or near–syncope as a result of impaired cardiac output due to ischemia–induced abnormalities of systolic or diastolic function. Subaortic obstruction, by increasing both left ventricular systolic and diastolic pressures, can lead to exactly the same constellation of symptoms.

Once it is recognized that several different pathophysiologic mechanisms can lead to the same set of symptoms, it becomes clear that therapeutic approaches must be directed not at the symptoms, which may have multiple causes, but at the specific mechanisms responsible for producing the symptoms in each individual patient. It also becomes clear why certain forms of treatment, which may work in some patients with a given symptom, may not work in other patients in whom the same symptom is caused by a different mechanism. For example, an operation (i.e., septal myotomy–myectomy or mitral valve replacement) would have a high probability of success if performed in a patient with a large gradient across the left ventricular outflow tract, but in whom intrinsic diastolic function is not markedly abnormal and in whom underlying mechanisms favoring the development of ischemia, other than LV outflow obstruction, are relatively unimportant. In contrast, operation would probably not exert a markedly salutary effect in the individual with only a mild to moderate gradient but in whom there is marked left ventricular hypertrophy contributing to major abnormalities in diastolic function and to the development of myocardial ischemia.

In summary, the pathophysiology of HCM is not only complicated, but varies enormously from one patient to another. It is only after the physician understands these diverse mechanisms and how they specifically relate to the symptoms experienced by the individual patient that the most effective approach to medical therapy can be devised.

References

1. Teare RD: Asymmetrical hypertrophy of the heart in young adults. Brit Heart J 20: 1–8, 1958.
2. Abbasi AS, MacAlpin RN, Eber LM, Pearce ML: Echocardiographic diagnosis of idiopathic hypertrophic cardiomyopathy without outflow obstruction. Circulation 46: 897–904, 1972.
3. Henry WL, Clark CE, Epstein SE: Asymmetric septal hypertrophy (ASH): echocardiographic identification of the pathognomonic anatomic abnormality of IHSS. Circulation 47: 225–233, 1973.
4. Abbasi AS, MacAlpin RN, Ebert LM, Pearce ML: Left ventricular hypertrophy diagnosed by echocardiography. N Engl J Med 289: 118–121, 1973.
5. Maron BJ, Gottdiener JS, Bonow RO, Epstein SE: Hypertrophic cardiomyopathy with unusual locations of left ventricular hypertrophy undetectable my M–mode echocardiography. Circulation 63 (No 2): 409–418, 1981.
6. Maron BJ, Gottdiener JS, Epstein SE: Patterns and significance of distribution of left ventricular hypertrophy in hypertrophic cardiomyopathy. A wide–angle, two–dimensional echocardiographic study of 125 patients. Am J Cardiol 48: 418–428, 1981.

7. Wigle ED, Adelman AG, Silver MD: Pathophysiological considerations in muscular subaortic stenosis. In: Hypertrophic obstructive cardiomyopathy. CIBA Foundation Study Group No 37, J and A Churchill London, 1971, pp 63–76.

8. Henry WL, Clark CE, Griffith JM, Epstein SE: Mechanism of left ventricular outflow obstruction in patients with obstructive asymmetric septal hypertrophy (idiopathic hypertrophic subaortic stenosis). Am J Cardiol 35: 337–345, 1975.

9. Bonow RO :Effects of calcium channel blocking agents on left ventricular diastolic function in hypertrophic cardiomyopathy and coronary artery disease. Am J Cardiol (in press).

10. Gaasch WH, Levine HJ, Quinones MA, Alexander JK: Left ventricular compliance: mechanisms and clinical implications. Am J Cardiol 38: 645–653, 1976.

11. Grossman W, Barry WH, Diastolic pressure–volume relations in the diseased heart. Federation Proc 39: 148–155, 1980.

12. St John Sutton MG, Tajik AJ, Gibson DG, Brown DJ, Seward JB, Guiliani ER: Echocardiographic assessment of left ventricular filling and septal and posterior wall dynamics in idiopathic hypertrophic subaortic stenosis. Circulation 57: 512–520, 1978.

13. Harmjanz D, Bottcher D, Schertlien G: Correlations of electrocardiographic pattern, shape of ventricular septum, and isovolumic relaxation time in irregular hypertrophic cardiomyopathy (obstructive cardiomyopathy). Brit Heart J 33: 928–937, 1971.

14. Hanrath P, Mathey DG, Siegert R, Bleifeld W: Left ventricular relaxation and filling in different forms of left ventricular hypertrophy: an echocardiographic study. Am J Cardiol 45: 15–23, 1980.

15. Bonow RO, Rosing DR, Bacharach SL, Green MV, Kent KM, Lipson LC, Maron BJ, Leon MB, Epstein SE: Effects of verapamil on left ventricular systolic function and diastolic filling in patients with hypertrophic cardiomyopathy. Circulation 64: 787–796, 1981.

16. Bonow RO, Frederick TM, Bacharach SL, Green MV, Goose PW, Maron BJ, Rosing DR: Atrial systole and left ventricular filling in patients with hypertrophic cardiomyopathy: effect of verapamil. Am J Cardiol 51: 1386–1391, 1983.

17. Bonow RO, Dilsizian V, Rosing DR, Indanpaan–Heikkila U, Epstein SE: Increased exercise tolerance by verapamil in hypertrophic cardiomypathy: relation to enhanced left ventricular diastolic filling. J Am Coll Cardiol (abstr). 3: 620, 1984.

18. Maron BJ, Epstein SE, Roberts WC: Hypertrophic cardiomyopathy and transmural myocardial infarction without significant atherosclerosis of the extramural coronary arteries. Am J Cardiol 43: 1086–1102, 1979.

19. McReynolds RA, Roberts WC: The intramural coronary arteries in hypertrophic cardiomyopathy. Am J Cardiol (abstr) 35: 154, 1975.

20. Rembert J, Kleimann L, Fedor J, Wechsler A, Greenfield J: Myocardial blood flow distribution in concentric left ventricular hypertrophy. J Glin Invest 62: 379, 1978.

21. Rakusan K: Quantitative morphology of capillaries of the heart: number of capillaries in animal and human hearts under normal and pathological conditions. Meth Achiev Exp Path 5: 272, 1971.

22. Aversano T, Klocke FJ: Effects of preload on diastolic coronary pressure–flow relationships. Circulation (abstr) 66: II–42, 1982.

23. Cannon RO, Rosing DR, Leon MB, Watson RM, Epstein SE: Influence of vasodilator reserve and left ventricular filling pressure on coronary blood flow in hypertrophic cardiomypathy. Submitted for publication.

24. Hernandez RR, Greenfield JC, McCall BW: Pressure–flow studies in hypertrophic subaortic stenosis. J Clin Invest 43: 401–407, 1964.

25. Criley JM, Lewis KB, White RI, Ross RS: Pressure gradients without obstruction: A new concept of 'Hypertrophic Subaortic Stenosis'. Circulation 32: 881–887, 1965.

26. Wilson WS, Criley JM, Ross RS: Dynamics of left ventricular emptying in hypertrophic subaortic stenosis: a cineangiographic and hemodynamic study. Am Heart J 73: 4–16, 1967.

27. Criley JM, Lennon PA, Abbasi AS, Balufuss AH: Hypertrophic cardiomyopathy. In: Levine HJ (ed), Clinical Cardiovascular Physiology. Grune and Stratton, New York, 1976, pp 771–827.

28. Murgo JP, Alter BR, Dorothy JF, Altobelli SA, McGrananhan GM: Dynamics of left ventricular ejection in obstructive and non–obstructive hypertrophic cardiomyopathy. J Clin Invest 66: 1369–1382, 1980.

29. Murgo JP: Does outflow obstruction exist in hypertrophic cardiomyopathy? N Engl J Med (ed) 307: 1008–1009, 1982.

30. Ross J Jr, Braunwald E, Gault JH, Mason DT, Morrow AG: The mechanisms of the intraventricular pressure gradient in idiopathic hypertrophic subaortic stenosis. Circulation 34: 558–578, 1966.

31. Wigle Ed, Marquis Y, Auger P: Muscular subaortic stenosis: initial left ventricular inflow tract pressure in the assessment of intraventricular pressure differences in man. Circulation 35: 1100–1117, 1967.

32. Epstein SE, Henry WL, Clark CG, Roberts WC, Maron BJ, Ferrans VJ, Redwood Dr, Morrow AG: Asymmetric septal hypertrophy. An Intern Med 81: 650–680, 1974.

33. Burchell HB: Pressure differences and obstruction of left ventricular outflow. Circulation (editorial) 34: 556–557, 1966.

34. Shah PM, Gramiak R, Kramer DH: Ultrasound location of left ventricular outflow obstruction in hypertrophic obstructive cardiomyopathy. Circulation 40: 3–11, 1969.

35. Popp RL, Harrison DC: Ultrasound in the diagnosis and evaluation of therapy of idiopathic hypertrophic subaortic stenosis. Circulation 40: 905Z8914, 1969.

36. Henry WL, Clark CE, Glancy DL, Epstein SE: Echocardiographic measurement of the left ventricular outflow gradient in idiopathic hypertrophic subaortic stenosis. N Engl J Med 288: 989–993, 1973.

37. Henry WL, Clark CE, Griffith JM, Epstein SE: Mechanism of left ventricular outflow obstruction in patients with obstructive asymmetric septal hypertrophy (idiopathic hypertrophic subaortic stenosis). Am J Cardiol 35: 337–345, 1975.

38. Gilbert BW, Pollick C, Adelman AG, Wigle Ed: Hypertrophic cardiomyopathy: subclassification by M–mode echocardiography. Am J Cardiol 45: 861–872, 1980.

39. Pierce GE, Morrow AG, Braunwald E: Idiopathic hypertrophic subaortic stenosis: III. Intraoperative studies of the mechanisms of obstruction and its hemodynamic consequences. Circulation 30 (suppl IV): 152–207, 1964.

40. Boughner DR, Schuld RL, Persaud JA: Hypertrophic obstructive cardiomyopathy. Assessment by echocardiographic and Doppler ultrasound techniques. Brit Heart J 37: 917–923, 1975.

41. Gardin Jm, Deabestani A, Glasgow GA, Butman S, Hughes C, Burn C, Henry WL: Doppler aortic blood flow studies in obstructive and non–obstructive hypertrophic cardiomypathy. (abstr) Circulation 66 (suppl II):·267, 1982.

42. Maron BJ, Gottdiener JS, Arce J, Rosing DR, Wesley YE, Epstein SE. Dynamic subaortic obstruction in hypertrophic cardiomyopathy: analysis by pulsed Doppler echocardiography. (Submitted for publication).

43. Maron BJ, Merrill WH, Freier PA, Kent KM, Epstein SE, Morrow AG: Long–term clinical course and symptomatic status of patients after operation for hypertrophic subaortic stenosis. Circulation 57: 1205–1213, 1978.

44. Morrow AG, Reitz BA, Epstein SE, Henry WL, Conkle DM, Itscoitz SV, Redwood DR: Operative treatment in hypertrophic subaortic stenosis: techniques, and the results of pre– and postoperative assessments in 83 patients. Circulation 52: 88–102, 1975.

45. Bigelow WG, Trimble AS, Wigle ED, Adelman AG, Felderhof CH: The treatment of muscular subaortic stenosis. J Thoral Cardiovasc Surg 68: 384–392, 1974.

46. Agnew TM, Barratt–Boyes BNC, Brandt PWT, Roche AHG, Lowe JB, O'Brien KP: Surgical resection in idiopathic hypertrophic subaortic stenosis with a combined approach through aorta and left ventricle. J Thorac Cardiovasc Surg 74: 307–316, 1977.

47. Reis RL, Hannah H, Carley JE, Pugh DM: Surgical treatment of idiopathic hypertrophic subaortic stenosis (IHSS) Postoperative results in 30 patients following ventricular septal myotomy and myectomy (Morrow procedure). Circulation 56 (suppl II): 128–132, 1977.
48. Beahrs MM, Tajik AJ, Seward JB, Giuliana ER, McGoon DC: Hypertrophic obstructive cardiomyopathy: 10–21 year follow-up after partial septal myectomy. Am J Cardiol 51: 1160–1166, 1983.
49. Spirito P, Maron BJ, Epstein SE: Morphologic determinants of hemodynamic state following ventricular septal myotomy–myectomy in patients with hypertrophic cardiomyopathy: M–mode and two–dimensional echocardiographic assessment. Circulation, in press.

Index of subjects